I0429799

Aromatherapy & Essential Oils for Beginners

Kimberly Jones

ISBN-13: 978-1500305260
ISBN-10: 150030526X

Disclaimer

The information specified throughout this book is provided for general information only, and should not be treated as a substitute for the medical advice of your own doctor, psychiatrist, medical counsellor or any other health care professional. Nothing contained on this book is intended to be for medical diagnosis or treatment. By following the instructions contained herein, the reader willingly assumes all risks in connection with such instructions. If you think you have a medical emergency, call your doctor immediately.

PROLOGUE

Contrary to popular belief, aromatherapy does not consist of merely buying a set of essential oils and then blending them at will for random use. Aromatherapy and proficient use of various forms of essential oils is an art that takes many years of diligent practice. However, due to the daily subjection to various forms of essential oils, everyone must now develop a practical approach to aromatherapy. The effects of this daily subjection to essential oils can be positive or negative, depending on your own uniqueness as a human being. Therefore, this guide is intended to help you obtain that necessary fundamental understanding of aromatherapy and essential oils. It is also designed to help you to become more consciously aware of other forms of olfactory stimulation that may be affecting your health.

In order to assist you in establishing a foundation for your ventures, this book presents you with a brief introduction and history of aromatherapy. It then moves on to cover such topics as types, forms and methods of extraction for essential oils. Next, this guide briefly takes you through explanations and samples of carrier oils, hot and cold oils and notes. Afterward, it provides you with a list of therapeutic benefits. Samples of essential oils used for obtaining those benefits accompany each of the listed benefits.

You will find examples of general uses and methods of diffusion throughout the entire book. However, specific examples of methods of diffusion for bath, body and room have also been included. Continuing to help you establish this foundation for your new skills as an aromatherapist, this guide also leads you through some hands-on experimentation.

After building a foundation to launch your exploration on, you will be ready to purchase essential oils. Therefore, I have included a short list of reputable online vendors. Of course, if you purchase any carrier or essential oil, you will then need to know how to store the oils properly. Thus, this guide will briefly touch upon that topic too. In the concluding sections of Part 1, you will find safety tips as well as a summary of the primary aromatherapy principles you need to know. Additionally, while revealing the most essential principles of aromatherapy, this book will address several common false assumptions made about essential oils and aromatherapy.

Part 2 is entirely devoted to sharing various types of beneficial recipes and formulas. Even though others have successfully used these recipes, I highly recommend that you do not attempt to use them prior to carefully reading Part 1. As is explained in Part 1, contrary to common belief, not every essential oil is suited to use by everyone. Each person has a unique reaction to every scent and what is beneficial to one person may harm another. Moreover, even the simplest, most beneficial essential oil can be harmful if improperly extracted or improperly used.

Nevertheless, once you have studied the more serious side of aromatherapy and essential oils, I hope you do take time to explore the lighter side of both. Aromatherapy and blending essential oils allows you to develop the artist, chef, scientist, chemist, researcher, teacher, healer, musician and inner child hidden within you. You will find yourself laughing over some experiments, while crying over others. For if nothing else, exploring the various uses of essential oils will be like taking a ride on an emotional and mental roller coaster. The journey will be filled with ups, downs and sudden, unexpected turns and twists. What makes it even more fun is that the experiences are not the same for any two people. So be sure you share and compare your unique experiences with others!

Chapter One: Aromatherapy Introduction and History

Aromatherapy, herbalism and essential oils have existed throughout the world for thousands of years. The healing, religious and rites of passage ceremonies of every known civilization included the use of aromatic plants in some form. In the past, aromatic plants and oils also served numerous other purposes, such as for culinary seasoning, camouflage, communication, marketing and for scenting cosmetic products. Throughout history, the use of essential oils saved many lives during plagues and other types of fatal epidemics.

Considered more valuable than any other type of asset, therapeutic essential oils and aromatic herbs also greatly enhanced their owners' lives in other ways in numerous ancient civilizations. Just owning essential oils in some past civilizations could turn an average person into a great political power.

Still used for all the same purposes in modern times, aromatic herbs and essential oils majorly affect our daily lives. However, nowadays, the use of olfactory stimuli has become such a natural part of our daily living that we are not typically consciously aware of the stimuli. We therefore tend to think of aromatherapy and essential oils as being new discoveries. In some ways, they are new discoveries for most humans.

In the past, only shamans, other tribal medicine men and women, priests, priestesses and doctors had a thorough knowledge of these herbs, plants and oils. The average citizens had to rely upon their religious leaders and healers to determine the right combination of essential oils and herbs to treat whatever ailed them. Fortunately, this is no longer true due to modern technology making this valuable information easily accessible to most literate human beings. Nevertheless, caution, discernment, advanced knowledge and some special skills are still necessary in order to use essential oils, aromatherapy and herbalism proficiently. Therefore, it is still best to seek out a professional herbalist, aromatherapist, naturopathic healer and/or medical doctor if you have any serious injuries or medical conditions that require advanced treatment.

Can Anyone Actually Define Aromatherapy?

An interesting fact is that no one can actually define the term "aromatherapy" in a way that is accepted by everyone. Although aromatherapy has been around for over ten thousand years, there is no one set concept as to what the term means. Therefore, several different definitions are given for aromatherapy. Some aroma experts insist that the term aromatherapy merely refers to the use of any pleasant aroma that enhances a living creature's life in some manner. This definition can include other uses too, such as pest control, beauty treatments and personal hygiene under the guise of aromatherapy.

Even gasoline and paint fumes would qualify as being aromatherapy under the auspices of this definition, since some people find them pleasant and uplifting. Some people even go to extra lengths to inhale these types of fumes in order to obtain a temporary euphoria. Nevertheless, medical professionals and research studies have proven that these types of olfactory stimulants can be very harmful to humans and other life forms when they are inhaled improperly.

Several medical dictionaries define aromatherapy as any aromatic aroma used as an alternative medical therapy treatment to cure or control an ailment. This definition would again include the use of other scent sources and non-therapeutic essential oils, as well as the essential oils that qualify as therapeutic. Due to this and the aforementioned definition, many people fail to distinguish the differences between herbalism and aromatherapy. Both, herbalism and aromatherapy make use of aromatic plants as alternative medical therapy treatments. Yet, several distinctions exist between the two, including methods of harvesting and plant usage. Herbalists typically use the plants themselves or utilize teas and infusions made from the plants. Aromatherapists typically just use the essential oils that have been extracted from the plants via distillation or expression.

However, yet other experts insist that aromatherapy is strictly the medical treatment of ailments via essential oils that qualify as being therapeutic. By this definition, not every aromatic plant, pleasant fragrance nor type or form of essential oil is used for aromatherapy. Nor are other uses for essential oils, such as pest control, considered as being aromatherapy.

You will have to decide for yourself what aromatherapy is. Nevertheless, this guide will cover topics from the perspective that all smells have an affect on people, whether it is a beneficial or harmful affect. It has been scientifically proven that humans automatically process olfactory stimuli via their nasal receptors and limbic systems. Certain chemical interactions occur when essential oils are ingested, inhaled or absorbed through or into the skin. Other affects are merely caused by the memories that are triggered by certain smells. Nonetheless, these memory-related affects still influence the person's mental, emotional, spiritual and physical well-being just as much as the chemical interactions do.

Chapter Two: What Qualifies as an Essential Oil?

Despite the disagreement as to what aromatherapy is, most experts do agree on what qualifies as an essential oil and its various forms. An essential oil is "a product made by distillation with either water or steam or by mechanical processing of citrus rinds or by dry distillation of natural materials. Following the distillation, the essential oil is physically separated from the water phase." At least, that is how the International Organization for Standardization (ISO) defines essential oils in their Vocabulary of Natural Materials (ISO/D1S9235.2). This is the most commonly accepted definition.

It is interesting to note that "essential oil" is actually a contraction of the original term used, which is "quintessential oil." The term, quintessential oil, derived from the Aristotelian ideology that assumes matter is composed of the elements of air, earth, fire, water and spirit. People believed that the distillation/evaporation process removed the plant's spirit or life force. Therefore, the harvesting of plants in ancient times was just as ceremonious as the extraction of essential oils. Each plant was carefully harvested by hand at certain times of the day and season.

Nowadays, people prefer to think that the plant matter has no life force or spirit. They believe the removed element is merely a physical mixture of complex chemicals. Modern chemists work hard to create concentrated formulas that replicate each plant's chemical properties. They then use these artificial substitutes in most consumer products rather than use the actual extracted oils

Perhaps thinking of plants as having life forces is better than thinking of them as merely being mixtures of chemical compounds. The fact remains that modern medicines and essential oils typically fail to induce the same therapeutic benefits as the same ingredients induced in ancient times. As modern technology finds its way into the distillation process, even more compounds find their way into and chemically adulterate the essential oils. This adulteration affects their therapeutic values.

Either way, in order for consideration as a "true" essential oil, utilizing physical means to isolate the fifth element by physical means is required. These physical means include steam, steam/water and water methods of distillation, expression (aka cold pressing) or maceration. Typically, maceration is utilized for extracting oil from a very limited number of plants, such as bitter almond, garlic and onion. Expression is typically used for removing the oil from citrus fruits.

Brief Introduction to Extraction Methods
Normally, the type of botanical material determines the method of extraction. Nonetheless, some exceptions exist, especially when utilizing CO2 extraction methods. The following is a list of commonly used extraction methods:

Distillation
This cost-effective process is the most popularly utilized method. It consists of converting the volatile essential oils into a vapor, then condensing the vapor back into a liquid. The essential oil is then separated from the water. Variations of the distillation method are water, steam, hydro diffusion, cohobation, rectification, water/steam and fractional distillation.

Expression
This cold pressed method of extraction is mostly used for squeezing oil from citrus peels, but can also be utilized for other plant materials. Variations of expression include scarification, sponge, ecuelle a piquer and machine abrasion.

Solvent Extraction

Rapidly becoming more popular as modern technology advances into the essential oil extraction industry, solvent extraction uses chemical solvents to separate the essential oils from their botanical materials. Both, absolutes and concretes are produced via solvent extraction methods. This method is frequently used when high heat or moisture can damage the essential oil. Methods of solvent extraction include maceration, enfleurage, solvent and hypercritical carbon dioxide (CO_2).

Hypercritical carbon dioxide extraction typically produces the finest quality of oil that is nearest to the original plant's constituency, but it is extremely expensive. Nonetheless many traditional aromatherapists are concerned that the use of solvents may alter the therapeutic value of the essential oil, and do not consider these types of oils to be "true" essential oils. Therefore, these types of essential oils are typically used for cosmetic products and perfumes instead of for aromatherapy treatments.

Importance of Knowing Methods of Extraction

Having a thorough knowledge of the aforementioned essential oil extraction methods is essential to your success with aromatherapy treatments and other essential oil applications. Thus, I highly encourage you to study these methods of extraction, even if you find the research boring. You may find websites similar to Aromatherapy Bible (http://www.aromatherapybible.com/extracting-essential-oils.html) very helpful in your research of essential oil extraction methods.

The method of extraction determines what form and quality the oil will have, which in turn determines what the best applications and methods of diffusion will be. Having this knowledge will also make you stop and think twice before you decide you want to make essential oils as a home-based enterprise.

For example, realizing that it takes distilling over 8 million blossoms to produce just 1 kilogram of jasmine oil would discourage most entrepreneurs. Can you imagine sitting at your kitchen table with your distiller and 8 million jasmine blossoms surrounding you? Think what it would be like to have to pick each one of those 8 million blossoms by hand! If you wish to make your own rose otto oil, you will need to distill 50-60 roses to extract 1 drop. To produce 1 kilogram of pure lemon oil, it takes 3,000 lemons.

Fortunately, most recipes and blends only require a few drops of each type of oil. In aromatherapy, less is better than more drops, as you can cause harmful affects by adding too much essence. Nevertheless, these samples should demonstrate that any pure essential oil that is highly therapeutic in nature is going to be relatively expensive. If it is not expensive, then it most likely is not truly a pure extract and therefore does not have as high of a therapeutic value as it would have otherwise. Nevertheless, there are some exceptions to this last statement.

Chapter Three: Cost, Quality, Forms and Types of Essential Oils

Cost and Quality Factors

As previously mentioned, the method of extraction influences the cost, quality, type and form of essential oils. Other factors that affect the quality, type, form and cost of essential oils are:

- **Location of Where Plant is Grown** -The climate, the altitude, the terrain and air/water pollutants highly influence the quality of the extract.

- **Season, Age of Plant and Timing of the Harvest** - Plants go through various growth stages that depend on the season of the year, the age of the plant and the time of day. If not harvested at the proper time, the extracted oil can be too potent or too weak.

- **Rarity of Botanical** - Oils extracted from rare, more exotic botanicals are likely to be much more expensive than oil extracted from more commonly found plant materials.

- **Distiller's and Country of Origin's Standards of Quality** - There are no set universal standards of quality or price, so the price and quality of essential oils can vary greatly among the various distillers and countries of origin.

Common Forms of Essential Oils

The type of botanical matter utilized also determines the method of extraction and what form the oil takes. The forms are commonly known as:

Absolute
Thick, heavy oil produced via removing the waxes and solvents form concretes through alcohol distillation. This process does not use water or heat, which highly damages delicate flowers during steam distillation processes. Absolutes are more concentrated, heavier and have stronger aromas than essential oils extracted by steam distillation. Due to the chemical residues of the solvents, some experts claim absolutes should not be used for aromatherapy. However, other experts claim that absolutes are not only safe but are also actually better to use for certain aromatherapy treatments. In my opinion, it depends on what benefits you want to obtain and your own level of sensitivity to the absolutes.

Adulterated
An essential oil that has had natural or artificial ingredients added to it after its distillation process was completed.

Concretes and Resinoids

The material extracted after the first stage of solvent distillation is completed. The mixture is usually too thick and heavy to be used for aromatherapy and requires special expertise to work with it. Concretes are waxy while Resinoids are resinous. Both are used in a wide range of industries.

Floral Water /Hydrosol /Hydroflorate / Distillates

The water that was used during a steam distillation process for extracting essential oils from flowers and other plants. The floral water has all the same properties as the whole plant or essential oil. However, it is milder and less concentrated than the essential oil from that plant. It is used in instances when essential oils would be too strong to utilize. Many laypersons commonly mistake floral water for essential oils, especially when first learning how to do essential oil extracting.

Fragrance Oils/Perfume Oils

Also known as aromatic oils, these types of oils are manufactured using synthetic materials. Although they replicate the fragrance of plants, they have none of the therapeutic qualities of the plant. They are used for flavoring foods and scenting cosmetic products.

Herbally Infused Oil

Oil made by infusing an herb with carrier oil, then removing the plant matter after the carrier oil has absorbed all the properties of the herb.

Neat
Essential oils that can be applied directly to the skin or ingested without use of a carrier oil or adulterant to dilute its potency or skin irritability potential.

Oleorresins
Oleorresins are the natural exudation of trees, such as elemi, Frankincense, gum and myrrh. They may also be extracted by acetone or alcohol. However, acetone extraction has been banned in most western countries.

Importance of Knowing the Various Forms of Essential Oils

Due to a widespread use of environmental fragrancing, people are exposed to huge amounts of olfactory stimuli via air conditioning diffusion in workplaces, restaurants, stores, hospitals, hotels and other places of business on a daily basis. People are also exposed to a wide range of absolutes, concretes, hydrosols and fragrance oils on a daily basis via various common consumer products. This exposure comes in the form of scented soap, laundry detergent, food flavorings and insecticide products. Most household cleaning products contain hydrosols, concretes or resinoids. Almost all personal hygiene products, cosmetic products and beverages contain some form of essential oil, hydrosols, esters, phenols, aldehydes or fragrance oil. Most products contain several of these olfactory stimuli.

Thus, since over-exposure to any scent may cause sensitization, it is essential that you learn how to identify and take control of the various olfactory stimuli that is affecting your health and well-being. The chapter on Safety Tips will provide you with ideas on how to avoid over-exposure to all forms of olfactory stimuli. For now, let us continue discussing the types of oils you will need to know about before purchasing any essential oil.

Types of Oils

Carrier Oils

Proper usage of most essential oils requires knowing how to choose the right oils, including the correct carrier oil. Carrier oils help to lessen the risk of skin irritation and to aid in the absorption of the essential oil. Most of the carrier oils (aka fixed oils or base oils) are cold pressed vegetable extractions from nuts and seeds. However, some use milk, egg whites or gels like aloe vera.

The most important thing to remember when choosing the carrier oil is that it has its own properties and scents. Some oils are best used for enhancing absorption through the skin while others enhance absorption into the skin. Some oils aid in making the essential oil easier to ingest or inhale. Here is a list of commonly used carrier oils and their properties:

• **Aloe Vera Gel** - Is used primarily for treating burns, cuts, wounds and in shower gels. Also is used for removing other types of carrier oils from sheets and can be taken internally.

•**Apricot Kernel Oil** - Is used to aid assimilation of food and is good for face oils and as base oil for personal blends. It is expensive, but leaves the skin silky smooth.

• **Borage Oil** - It is expensive and needs to be kept refrigerated, but is good for all skin types and works as an anti-aging agent. Borage oil is very good for use in massage oil blends. However, it should never make up more than 3%-5% of the blend.

• **Canola Oil** - It is very light and has a long shelf life. Since it is readily absorbed, canola oil makes a great base for massage oil blends.

• **Castor Oil** - This oil activates the immune system and boosts energy to areas that need it. It can be used for children and is good for congestion and Edgar Cayce packs.

• **Grape-Seed Oil** - This light oil penetrates quickly and will sometimes stain. It only has a slight smell, which makes it good for facial oils. Typically, it is used for cleaning and toning oily skin.

• **Hazelnut Oil** - This deep penetrating oil contains Vitamin A and nourishes the skin. It is used as a light astringent and circulation stimulant.

• **Jojoba Oil** - This emollient oil does not get rancid and is quickly absorbed. It is primarily used for hair care, dissolving sebum and lightening up other oils.

• **Sesame Oil** - This oil has an odor and color, but it is good for filtering sunrays. It is also good for treating psoriasis and eczema.

• **Sweet Almond Oil** - Used primarily as a base for massage oils, this oil is rich in proteins and does not have much of a smell. It provides excellent protection for the skin and is emollient. Sweet almond oil is used for relieving itching, mosquito bites and measles. However, it does have a tendency to go rancid.

• **Wheat Germ Oil** - This anti-scarring, anti-oxidant oil is rich in vitamins, especially Vitamin A. It is good for dry skin and is typically added to blends and massage oils to promote firmness and elasticity in skin.
Numerous other oils also make fine base oils. However, most mineral oils are not used as carrier oils due to their tendency to block the absorption of the volatile essential oils. Many people choose to blend the carrier oils in order to increase the therapeutic benefits.

A sample of a specially blended carrier oil is one that contains canola oil (60%), jojoba oil (20%), castor oil (10%), evening primrose oil (5%), borage oil (5%), Vitamin E (1 1000 IU capsule), and wheat germ oil (1 "blop"). As you can see, even making special carrier oils can be complicated. It is highly recommended that you do not attempt to blend more than 2-3 carrier oils until you have become familiar with each type of oil. This also brings up the point that you should never blend more than 5-6 essential oils in a single formula. As a lay aromatherapist, you should not blend more than 2-3 essential oils, and that is only after you have thoroughly explored each of the ingredients individually.

As you experiment with the carrier and essential oils, let the scientist and researcher in you come out by keeping a chart that includes the exact recipe you used and your reactions to it. Also, record the reaction of pets and anyone else that has been exposed to the formula. Any chef will tell you how hard it is to remember even the simplest recipe if you forget to write it down. It is quite easy to forget which types of oil and how many drops of oil were used once you have completed making a new blend, especially if you become distracted during the blending process. It is also quite easy to forget what you liked or disliked about an oil or fragrance due to there being over 700 essential oils, with new blends coming out on the market daily.

If you need a reminder as to why it is important to keep records, simply go into your kitchen and mix several spices and other ingredients together. Do not record what your mixture contains. Then go back and attempt to make an exact replica one week later, or even just a few days later. For that matter, try to make an identical copy of the mixture just three or four hours later. Make sure that you have someone else record the exact ingredients and the amounts added though. That way you can compare the ingredients and amounts and recognize in what manner you altered the mixture during the replication process.

Is it Hot or Cold oil?

The most important thing to remember when making your own blends is that essential oils are either hot or cold oils. Hot oils are not absorbed through the skin via the carrier oil as cold oils are. Therefore, any time you use hot oils, you must adulterate them with cold oils as well as with carrier oils. The shape, color and therapeutic qualities of the plant the oil is extracted from will help you know whether it is hot or cold oil. For instance, oil from a red flower or that is used to treat the reproductive system is likely to be a hot oil. The location and conditions that the plant is grown in, as well as which part of the plant produces the essential oil is also indicative of its hot or cold nature. For instance, essential oil taken from the reproductive system of the plant is likely to be hot. The method of extraction will also help you recognize which type it is and what is the best way to integrate it into your special blends.

Is it a Top, Middle or Base Note?

Another matter of importance when making your own blends is knowing whether the oil is a top, middle or base note. In music composition, the composer must take into consideration the sounds and every effect that each instrument or voice is capable of producing. If the notes, voices or instruments clash, then the musical piece is disruptive, unpleasant and difficult to listen to due to the disharmony. If one instrument drowns out the sounds made by another instrument, then the listener does not hear a part of the music.

With aromatherapy, the therapist must make every effort to make the blend of carrier and essential oils just as harmoniously as if it were a musical composition. If improperly blended, the essential oils may lose their therapeutic benefits. An improper choice could cause an oil to nullify or counteract sine some other oil or one scent could overpower another scent. Thus, each essential oil is categorized as a top, middle or base note as well as by its therapeutic value, constituents and botanical family.

Top Notes

Top note oils are like the flute section of an orchestra or the soprano section of a choir. They should make up 1%-5% of the total blend. They are the oils that personify the blend, as they are the first thing you smell. Top notes are very volatile, evaporate quickly and are very aromatic. They are sharp and extremely penetrating whether they are hot or cold essential oils. Top notes are used for brightening a blend, stimulating and clearing your mind and uplifting your energy.

Examples of top notes are Bergamot, cinnamon, clove, all citrus oils, lemongrass, neroli, Petitgrain and thyme. Some of these oils can be used liberally, while others must be used sparingly. For instance, bergamot and Petitgrain can be used liberally, while all citrus oils, neroli and clove should be used sparingly. Most of the essential oils extracted from fruits and flowers are top notes. However, some can be used as top or middle notes, like tangerine oil.

Middle Notes
As any composer knows, music does not sound right in monotones. Therefore, the composer creates harmony parts to go along with those sopranos voices. The middle note oils are like the heart of the orchestra or choir and should make up 60%-80% of the blend. Middle notes include the groups of oils known as enhancers and equalizers and can include oils from the top note and base note groups. They enhance the blend, giving it a warm, soft

and mellow body while equalizing the blend by smoothing out the sharp edges. Middle notes have their own pleasant fragrances and have enough personality to modify the blend, yet they do not overpower the other oils. The middle notes create the harmony of the blend, and provide balance physically and energetically. They help to soothe your mind and body. Middle note oils are typically extracted from leaves, stems and flowers. Examples of middle notes are chamomile, geranium, lavender, marjoram and rosewood.

Although the enhancers can make up to 50% of the total blend, each of the individual enhancer oils should only make up to 15% of the blend. Examples of blend enhancers are bergamot, cedarwood, clary sage, geranium, jasmine, lavender, lemon, lime, litesea cubeba, myrrh, neroli, Palmarosa, rose, sandalwood, spruce and ylang ylang. The equalizers can make up to 50% of the total blend. Common blend equalizers are rosewood and wild Spanish marjoram. Orange and tangerine are typically used for blending citruses, spices and florals, while fir and pine is typically used for improving blends of myrtaceae or coniferesae.

Base Notes
Although music sounds good with just the soprano and alto voices singing or playing in

harmony, the composer knows it sounds even better if deeper voices or lower-voiced instruments are added in to keep the sopranos and altos in sync. Therefore, the base notes are like the deep-voiced instruments in the orchestra or bass singers in a choir. They give the blend a deep, warm quality and act as fixatives by reducing the top notes' rate of evaporation. Base notes are typically earthy scented essential oils that are derived from resins, roots and woods. The base notes typically are used for treating anxiety, insomnia and stress, as well as used for calming and spiritually grounding a person.

Base note oils are deep, intense, thus drawing into the skin and affecting the chakras. They typically smell stronger on the skin than they do in the bottle, so they should be used sparingly. Thus, base notes should only make up 10% of the total blend, with each of the base oils individually making up 5% of the blend. Examples of base notes are cedarwood, clary sage, Frankincense, myrrh, sandalwood and vertver.

The base note oils also include a group of oils known as blend modifiers due to their ability to alter the overall smell of the blend. These oils should be used even more sparingly (1%-3%) than the aforementioned base notes. Although they liven up a flat blend, they can easily kill the blend if even just one drop too many is added. Examples of blend modifiers are blue chamomile, cistus, cinnamon, cloves, patchouli, peppermint, thyme and ylang ylang.

How to Combine the Notes Harmoniously

Now that you understand what the notes are, it is time to learn how to combine them in a harmonious manner. The most recommended way to make a blend is to add one drop at a time. First, pick out the top, middle and base notes that most appeal to your own senses. As you should have inferred from reading about the various notes, each note is meant to affect a specific part of a person, while still interacting with the other oils to address the person's overall needs. Thus, before choosing any oils, you must take into consideration that person's overall homeostasis and then worry about the individual health issues. The primary purpose of using aromatherapy is to establish a total state of well-being with smells and essential oils.

Once you have assessed yourself as a whole person and evaluated your health issues, then choose one top note and start with one drop of it on the tip of a cotton swab. Smell it. Then add one drop of your chosen middle note to another cotton swab and take a whiff of it. Take a whiff of the two cotton swabs before adding the base note to a third cotton swab. Once you have smelled all three scents simultaneously, decide what else needs to be added, whether it be more drops of the same three oils or a different combination of oils. Be sure to test for negative reactions to every ingredient prior to mixing the final blend. The chapter on safety tips includes instructions on how to test for negative reactions.

Chapter Four: Terminology for Therapeutic Benefits

By now, you are probably to the point where you want to do some type of hands-on experimentation with essential oils rather than just read about them. It is probably quite tempting to skip the rest of Part 1 of this guide and go on to Part 2 to find the recipes and formulas that might relate to your specific needs. Nevertheless, there is still much more information you need to know before playing around with essential oils and trying out the formulas. For instance, you will need to know the terminology used for describing the various therapeutic benefits. Therefore, I propose a compromise - I let you experiment with aromatherapy via aromas you can probably find in your kitchen spice rack and then you get back to studying Part 1 of this guide before venturing into Part 2.

Are you ready for the experiment? Then go into your kitchen and find some sage, mint, coffee grounds and/or cocoa. If you are feeling a bit overwhelmed and need a bit of mental clarity, then rub some of the sage on your hands. Just take an occasional whiff of the sage as you finish reading this guide. By the way, this works well if you have to take a tough exam at school or stay focused for long periods while at work.

If you feel a bit spacey or flighty, then take a good whiff of the coffee grounds. However, do not drink a cup of coffee! Research has revealed that one cup of coffee can lower a healthy person's energy hertz from the normal range of 62-68 GHz to just 52 GHz in about 22 seconds. The coffee will keep the person feeling low on energy for three days, unless immediately given an essential oil energy stimulant.

If you feel a bit nervous or anxious, then either place the mint nearby or ingest it if it is in an edible form. The cocoa aroma will brighten your mood and relax you if you are feeling a bit down or stressed. However, each person is unique and you may have to find some other spices or aromas around your house to calm your nerves and clear your head. You should eventually take the time to go on a scavenger hunt throughout your home and try to identify each scent that is affecting you, your family and any visitors to your home. For instance, some of the aromas found in your kitchen may be stimulating or suppressing people's appetites. Some may be causing kidney, liver or bladder ailments. Others may be causing skin irritation or may be causing depression or sadness. Yet other aromas may be uplifting your spirits or providing you with a source of unexplained energy.

Anyway, now that you have finished the experiment, let us continue with broadening your knowledge of essential oils and aromatherapy. Here is an abridged list of the therapeutic benefits provided through essential oils, along with examples of which oils offer them:

Analgesic
Pain reliever – Examples:

- *Basil*
- *Bergamot*
- *Eucalyptus radiata*
- *Cardamom*
- *Geranium*

- *Bay (Laurel)*
- *Black Pepper*
- *Chamomile (German and Roman)*
- *Fir*
- *Ginger*

- *Juniper berry*
- *Peppermint*
- *Tea tree*

- *Niaouli*
- *Rosemary*

Antibacterial/Anti-infectious/Antiseptic
Destroys bacteria, helps to prevent and/or fight infections - Examples:

- *Basil*
- *Citronella*
- *Eucalyptus (citriodora and globulus)*
- *Lemon*
- *Lemon verbena*
- *Myrtle*

- *Cinnamon*
- *Geranium*
- *Lavender*
- *Lemongrass*
- *Melissa*
- *Pine*

Antidepressant

Brightens dark moods, relieves depression and sadness - Examples:

- *Basil*
- *Bay (Laurel)*
- *Geranium*
- *jasmine*
- *Lemon*
- *Litsea cubeba*
- *Patchouli*
- *Rosemary*

- *Bergamot*
- *Clary sage*
- *Grapefruit*
- *Lavender*
- *Lemongrass*
- *Orange (sweet)*
- *Rose*
- *ylang ylang*

Anti-fungal

Fungus growth inhibitor - Examples:

- *Basil*
- *Chamomile (German)*

- *Clary sage*
- *Litsea cubeba*
- *Patchouli*
- *Ravensara*
- *Spearmint*
- *Tea tree*
- *Geranium*
- *Marjoram (sweet)*
- *Peppermint*
- *Rosemary*
- *Spruce*

Anti-inflammatory

Reduces and/or prevents inflammation and relieves pain from inflammation - Examples:

- *Basil*
- *Chamomile (German)*
- *Fennel (sweet)*
- *Geranium*
- *Lavender*
- *Litsea cubeba*
- *Marjoram (sweet)*
- *Niaouli*
- *Patchouli*
- *Peppermint*
- *Ravensara*
- *Rose*
- *Rosemary*
- *Spearmint*
- *Spruce*
- *Tea tree*

Antispasmodic

Alleviates spasms in voluntary and involuntary muscles - Examples:

- *Basil*
- *Black Pepper*
- *Chamomile (German , Roman)*
- *Cinnamon*
- *Clary sage*
- *Cypress*
- *Eucalyptus radiata*
- *Fennel (sweet)*
- *Geranium*
- *jasmine*
- *Juniper berry*
- *Lavender*
- *Lemon*
- *Mandarin*

Astringent

Firms tissue and organs; reduces discharges and secretions - Examples:

- *Cedarwood (Atlas)*
- *Cypress*
- *Eucalyptus radiata*
- *Frankincense*
- *Geranium*
- *Juniper berry*
- *Lemon*
- *Lemongrass*
- *Litsea cubeba*
- *Patchouli*
- *Peppermint*
- *Rose*
- *Rosemary*
- *Vetiver*

Calming
Soothing, relaxing, relieves anxiety and nervous tension - Examples:

- *Basil*
- *Geranium*
- *Lavender*
- *Marjoram (sweet)*

- *Clary sage*
- *Juniper berry*
- *Lemon*
- *Pine*

Carminative

Relieves intestinal gas pain and distention; promotes peristalsis - Examples:

- *Basil*
- *Bergamot*
- *Cardamom*

- *Bay (Laurel)*
- *Black Pepper*
- *Chamomile (German and Roman)*

- *Fennel (sweet)*

- *Frankincense*

- *Ginger*
- *Lavender*
- *Lemongrass*
- *Mandarin*

- *Orange (sweet)*

- *Rosemary*

- *Juniper berry*
- *Lemon*
- *Litsea cubeba*
- *Marjoram (sweet)*

- *Peppermint*

- *Thyme*

Cephalic
Treatment for the head, typically clearing and stimulating - Examples:

- *Basil*
- *Peppermint*
- *Spearmint*

- *Cardamom*
- *Rosemary*

Cicatrisant

Regenerative for skin cells, resists scarring - Examples:

- *Bergamot*

- *Eucalyptus radiata*

- *Geranium*

- *Lemon*

- *Patchouli*

- *Rosemary*

- *Tea tree*

- *Chamomile (German)*

- *Frankincense*

- *Lavender*

- *Niaouli*

- *Rose*

- *Spearmint*

- *Thyme*

Decongestant

Reduces nasal mucus production and swelling - Examples:

- *Chamomile (German)*
- *Clary sage*
- *Eucalyptus radiata*
- *Fennel (sweet)*
- *Geranium*
- *Grapefruit*
- *Juniper berry*
- *Lavender*
- *Lemon*
- *Mandarin*
- *Marjoram (sweet)*
- *Niaouli*
- *Orange (sweet)*
- *Patchouli*
- *Peppermint*
- *Ravensara*
- *Rose*
- *Rosemary*

Diuretic

Helps with activity in kidney and bladder and increases urination - Examples:

- *Cardamon*
- *Cypress*
- *Fennel (sweet)*
- *Geranium*
- *Lavender*
- *Marjoram (sweet)*
- *Pine*
- *Thyme*

- *Cedarwood (Atlas)*
- *Eucalyptus radiata*
- *Frankincense*
- *Grapefruit*
- *Mandarin*
- *Patchouli*
- *Rosemary*

Expectorant
Promotes discharge of phlegm and mucus from the lungs and throat - Examples:

- *Basil*
- *Cardamom*
- *Eucalyptus radiata*
- *Frankincense*
- *Marjoram (sweet)*
- *Peppermint*
- *Ravensara*
- *Thyme*

- *Bay (Laurel)*
- *Cedarwood (Atlas)*
- *Fennel (sweet)*
- *Ginger*
- *Niaouli*
- *Pine*
- *Tea tree*

Immunostimulant
Stimulates functioning of the immune system - Examples:

- *Cypress*

- *Frankincense*

- *Niaouli*
- *Patchouli*
- *Spruce*
- *Tea tree*

Sedative
Calms and tranquilizes a person by lowering the functional activity of an organ or body part - Examples: Bergamot, cedarwood (Atlas), Chamomile (German and Roman), clary sage, Frankincense, jasmine, lavender, lemongrass, mandarin, marjoram (sweet), orange (sweet), patchouli, rose, vetiver and ylang ylang.

Stimulant
Increases functional activity of specific organ or system - Examples:

- *Basil*
- *Cardamom*
- *Cinnamon*
- *Fir*
- *Ginger*
- *Grapefruit*
- *Juniper berry*
- *Litsea cubeba*
- *Niaouli*
- *Peppermint*

- *Rosemary*
- *Tea tree*
- *Spearmint*
- *Thyme*

Tonic
Strengthens and restores vitality - Examples:

- *Basil*
- *Bergamot*
- *Juniper berry*
- *Litsea cubeba*
- *Niaouli*
- *Ravensara*
- *Rosemary*
- *Bay (Laurel)*
- *Black Pepper*
- *Lemon*
- *Marjoram (sweet)*
- *Pine*
- *Rose*
- *Spearmint*

- *Spruce*
- *Thyme*

- *Vetiver*

Did you notice that many of the oils in the aforementioned list are also from the same plants as the spices and foods you found in your kitchen? Did you also notice that many of the oils could be used for several purposes? I hope that you noticed how many of the oils used for a specific therapeutic benefit all came from the same botanical family or came from the same category of constituents. Many of the oils came from the same parts of the plants, i.e. roots, petals or stems. It is important to remember that you can sometimes substitute oils from the same botanical family or category of constituents when you are lacking or cannot afford a particular essential oil. It is also a good idea to remember that many of the items in your kitchen can be used as pinch-hitters in your first-aid kit because they do contain some form of essential oil, even if it is not at the therapeutic grade level. For instance, you can make a paste out of meat tenderizer and water to reduce the pain and draw out the stinger from a wasp or bee sting.

More Terms

Numerous other terms are also applied to the effects of essential oils and aromatherapy. Some other terms you may need to know when choosing your oils for use in your daily life are:

• Anti-pyretic - disperses heat, reduces fevers

• Anti-viral - prevents viruses from growing

• Emetic - causes vomiting

•Emmenagogue - aids in promoting and regulating menstruation

• Emollient - smoothes, softens and protects the skin

•Haemostatic - stops the flow of blood, especially as an astringent that stops internal bleeding or hemorrhaging

• Hypotensive - lowers high blood pressure

• Laxative - promotes bowel movements

• Mucolytic - breaks down pulmonary mucous

The list of terms could become quite long, so I will end it here. However, I do highly encourage you to become familiar with the terminology used in aromatherapy. You will find that many terms are also used in the various medical fields as well as in labeling on various consumer products. The best way to learn these terms and which oils to use is to purchase a chart from a reputable company that manufacture essential oils, such as Young Living Oils or doTerra. However, many websites allow you to make a printed copy of their charts without paying any fees.

These usage charts come in a wide variety of styles. Some charts classify the essential oils by name, and then give their therapeutic benefits, other qualities and methods of diffusion. Other charts list the condition first, and then list all the essential oils that can be used to treat that condition. There are also charts that start out with the methods of diffusion, and then list which oils are best diffused in that manner, followed by the benefits each oil provides when diffused in that manner.

You will have to decide which type of chart works best for you. You may want to make up your own chart as you experiment with the oils. Everyone has a unique response. We each respond in a unique manner to everything our senses intercept. Our actions and reactions are all based on what experiences we remember having in the past as we see, hear, smell, taste and feel things in the present. Fortunately, or perhaps unfortunately, no two living creatures have the exact memories. Individuals also have their own unique energy pattern that interacts with the energy patterns of everything that surrounds them. Therefore, that which one person considers to be calming another person may find to be stimulating. Thus, it really does not matter how someone else responds to a particular aroma, essential oil or health treatment. It only matters how you as an individual respond to them.

Chapter Five: General Methods of Diffusing Essential Oils

So far, you have gained a basic knowledge of the history, types and forms of oils, what purposes they serve, and how to mix a simple blend of oils. Next, you will learn how to diffuse the oil via various methods of application. Having so many options available to you may make choosing a method of diffusion very difficult for you.

However, the methods of diffusion usually depend on the intended purpose, the particular essential oils chosen and personal preferences. For instance, wound care is generally done topically in order to address the wound directly. Mood setting, even though it can be accomplished by topical means, is generally done via a room diffuser because it gets faster results.

When choosing a method, you should remember that there are primarily three ways that the oils enter a person's body. Thus, all the methods of oil application can be categorized by these three ways of entrance. These ways are inhalation (via nose), internally (via mouth or rectum) or topically (via skin). Each of these three categories includes several application methods. For instance, essential oils can be topically applied in ways that enhance absorption into the skin or that enhances absorption through the skin.

Inhalation Applications

Inhalation methods normally highly dilute essential oils in order to make it easier for them to be absorbed by the limbic system, brain, blood system and various organs of the body. Thus, inhalation methods typically elicit quick responses to whatever oil is being diffused. These inhalation methods are the best diffusion method for oils that are typically irritating to the skin. It is also the best method of diffusion for environmental fragrancing or affecting several people simultaneously. For instance, if you wanted to keep all the family members calm during an important discussion, you could use a room diffuser to disperse basil or another calming essential oil into the air.

Inhalation methods include:
Using a Heat Diffuser
This entails placing essential oils into a device that evaporates the oils via heat. Some require using water in the device to create the evaporation process.

Using a Cold Diffuser
This method is the dispersment of the oils into the air without the use of heat. You can do

this adding a few drops of essential oil to cotton balls and then placing the cotton balls in an air conditioning vent or in front of an electric fan. You can also do this by adding a few drops of essential oils to a cloth that has been dampened with water and then hanging the cloth up in front of an air vent or wherever else the air circulates.

Using Dry Evaporation
This involves placing several drops of essential oil on a tissue or cotton ball and then placing in the immediate area of the person being treated. This lets the essential oils simply evaporate into the air, with the potency being determined by the person's proximity to the cotton ball or tissue.

Using a Spray
This method consists of combining drops of essential oils with a water-based solution in a spray bottle. You simply place the oil in the solution, shake the bottle and then spray the mixture into the air. This method is typically used for deodorizing the air or setting a mood. However, if you forget to shake the bottle, you will end up just spraying water into the air. Most essential oils are not water-soluble.

Using Steam
In this method, the essential oils are added to a container of steaming water. The steam

quickly evaporates the oils so you have to act fast. After placing the oils in the steaming water, hold a towel over your head as you bend your head toward the container and breathe deeply. Since this method is very potent, it is essential for you to keep your eyes closed during the treatment. No one should use more than 1-2 drops of oil, and children under 7 years old should not be exposed to the essential oils in this manner. If a child is older than 7 years old, and chooses this method, then he or she should wear swimming goggles or some other type of sealed eye protection.

Cold diffusion methods are now considered safer and more effective than the heated diffusion methods. This is due to the way heat alters the chemicals in the essential oils and creates toxic compounds. However, there are some exceptions to this theory and some essential oils must be diffused via heat or steam. In all circumstances, it is best not to burn essential oils, as it can create carcinogenic compounds. For the best results, follow the instructions given on the label. If you are still unsure which method to use, then consult an experienced aromatherapist.

Internal Applications

There are two primary ways essential oils are administered internally. One way is via ingestion through the mouth. The other way is via suppositories placed in the rectum. Anyone who does not have a thorough knowledge of essential oils should use neither method. Reading books and experimenting with a few essential oils does not qualify you as an expert on essential oils. Therefore, it is highly recommended that you do not take any essential oils internally without supervision from a licensed healthcare practitioner.

Topical Applications

Topical applications cover a wide range of methods and provide you with the most options based on personal preferences. This is because essential oils can be added to many types of products. Here is a list of some of those topical options:

• **Added to massage products** - Includes creams, oils, lotions and gels.

• **Added to bath products** - Includes bath water, bath oils, bath salts, shower gels, body washes, soap, shampoo and hair conditioner

• **Added to a gargle/mouth rinse** - Be sure you do not swallow any! Just rinse your mouth with the solution and then spit it out.

• **Added to spa treatments** - Includes body wraps, facials, hand lotions, hand creams, manicures and pedicures.

• **Added to compresses** - This includes cold and hot packs

Added to other types of creams, lotions, gels, ointments and liniments -
Essential oils can be added directly to some unscented mixtures. They may have to be

diluted before adding in to other mixtures. Diluted oils can even be used for treating wounds by placing a drop of the adulterated oil directly on the bandage.

Essential oils may also be used in acupressure treatments, shiatsu treatments and feng shui. The most important thing to remember when using essential oils topically is that most of the oils should not be applied directly to the skin. Nor should an essential oil be used to cover a large portion of the body unless it is properly adulterated with carrier oil and cold oil.

Chapter Six: Specific Samples of Diffusion - Body, Bath and Room

By now, you are ready for another hands-on experiment. Therefore, if you already have some essential oils, here are some specific samples of diffusing them for the body, bath and room.

For Body: Simply add about 80 drops of essential oils to an 8 oz. bottle of unscented body lotion. Shake well, and apply the lotion directly to your skin, using circular motions. Use a floral scent for relaxation, or wood scent for centering. If you want to entice the opposite sex, then use a musky scent.

For Bath: Combine one part baking soda, two parts Epsom salts and three parts sea salt. Then set aside this mixture, which is known as a bath base. When you take your next bath, add 5-6 drops of true lavender essential oil to two tablespoons of bath base. Then mix the combined mixture into the bath water just before you enter the tub.

Remember that essential oils are not water-soluble, so the oil will float on top of the water and be absorbed by any skin that touches the oil. You will want to remember not to get the bath water in your eyes or to get any of the essential oils in your eyes while bathing. You may also want to remember that this method allows the essential oil to be inhaled as well as absorbed through the skin.

For Room: Freshen the air by combining 20 drops of lavender, 10 drops of lemon, 6 drops of bergamot, 5 drops of lime, and 5 drops of grapefruit with 1 cup of distilled water in a spray bottle. Shake well and then spray the room until the air smells fresher.

If you do not have your essential oils yet, then try these methods out:

For Body - Pick as many flowers from your garden as you can and boil them in a pan of water on top the stove. While the mixture is cooling off a bit, strip off your clothing and apply a carrier oil or unscented massage oil or gel to your skin. Wipe off any excess oil, lotion or gel. Then dip a sheet in the floral water. You want the mixture to be as hot as you can bear it. Wring the sheet out so that it is just damp and not soaking wet. Next, tightly wrap your body with the sheet. Then cover up with a warmed blanket, sheet or towel to hold in the heat from the body wrap. It is best to find a waterproof area to lie down in while wrapped up this way. You can use a shower curtain or vinyl tablecloth to cover your bed or a couch if you want to be more comfortable. It is also best to have a friend help you with the wrapping and covering you up. Stay wrapped up this way for 10-30 minutes or until you get uncomfortable. You can repeat this procedure up to three times in one session.

For Bath - Follow the steps in the previous paragraph, except dip a washcloth in the floral water instead of a sheet. Then just use the washcloth to bathe your body. You may also try mixing some of the floral water in with your tub water and just soak in the tub for a little while. If you choose to mix the floral water with your tub water, remember to add it to a bath base blend first. Although floral water is milder than pure essential oils, it can still cause skin irritation when

For Room - Find some pleasant spices or citrus juices in your kitchen. Apply them to cotton balls and then set the cotton balls in the air vents of your home or in an area of the room where there is air circulation occurring. Alternatively, simply place the cotton balls nearby so you can get a good whiff of the aromas.

Chapter Seven: Becoming Consciously Aware of Hidden Affects of Olfactory Stimuli

Now that you have been through these experiments with essential oils and scents found in your home, it is time to think about what you have learned. Have you noticed how much the aromas and spices in your kitchen can be used for other applications besides culinary seasonings? You learned that most foods, seasonings and beverages have some form of essential oil in them. Although these do not offer the same quality of therapeutic benefits as pure essential oils offer, they do affect your overall well-being in some manner.

You must also become more consciously aware of the olfactory stimuli that are in all the other consumer products you use. Moreover, you must become consciously aware of environmental fragrancing and the olfactory stimuli that surround you outside your home. As was mentioned in chapter four, you most likely have not associated these affects with the smells that are causing the affects. It is highly important that you take the time to do so.

These pleasant aromas and bad odors are not just affecting you in the most obvious ways, such as causing an allergic reaction or headache. They are also affecting you in hidden ways. Various research studies have revealed that many humans, especially those living in first-world countries, are losing their sense of smell. According to Cardiff University's website (http://www.cf.ac.uk/biosi/staffinfo/jacob/A nosmia/anosmia.html), approximately 2,000,000 Americans suffer from smell and taste disorders. This is considered an underestimated number since many people do not seek medical treatment for smell and taste disorders.

This may not seem important, but the truth is that humans rely on their sense of smell for numerous reasons. We rely on our sense of smell for survival, as it protects us from dangers such as fires, predatory animals and food poisoning. The sense of smell also directly affects the limbic system, communication, sexual activities, emotions, mental attitudes and the sense of taste. Smelling disorders can also be signs of other illnesses, such as Alzheimer's disease, Parkinson's disease, schizophrenia and dementia. Smelling disorders can also lead to low self-esteem, social alienation and depression. Despite how old the human race is, researchers are just beginning to discover how important the sense of smell is to humans.

Nevertheless, my point is that humans need to protect their senses of smell. Thus, you must be on guard against the constant bombardment of olfactory stimuli. You must also be aware of how you are contributing to that bombardment of smells. Everyone creates some of these smells naturally while creating other smells by artificial means. Nevertheless, we can never truly know how the smells we create or wear are affecting someone else. We simply have no way of knowing what memory will be triggered by the various smells. Nor do we truly know what effect some random smell will have on us as we venture through life, since we do not consciously know what memories our brains have associated with each smell our noses intercepted. Still, each of us must make an effort to take control of the smells that enhance our lives or harms us.

However, until you experiment with the various scents, you cannot truly take control over those emotional, mental, physical and spiritual affects that olfactory stimuli have on you on a more conscious level. This, in turn, means that you cannot reap the most rewards in your interpersonal relationships until you become aware of how these stimulants are affecting you and other people. Therefore, I highly encourage you to keep accurate records and actively experiment with all types of smells and not just those from essential oils. However, you will need to know some safety tips if you are going to be experimenting with the various oils and aromas. So let us continue on to the chapter on safety tips.

Chapter Eight: Safety Tips and Cautionary Warnings

As with everything else in life, essential oils must be used cautiously. Contrary to common myths and erroneous beliefs, not all essential oils are meant to be used by every person. Numerous "natural" or "organic" essential oils and herbs are toxic and are not safe to use. It is a false assumption that everything that is natural or organic is healthy for you. It is also a false assumption that what is good for one person must be good for everyone else. Thus, each of the essential oils comes with its own set of contraindications for use. The most common of these contraindications are:

Asthma

People with asthma should avoid camphor, marjoram, oregano, rosemary and yarrow.

Allergies

Everyone should test a small amount of oil on an area with sensitive skin (i.e. the inside of an elbow or upper arm) for 30 minutes prior to using it in other areas. Keep vegetable oil handy in case you start to have a reaction. People with known allergies to certain plants should avoid oils derived from those plants.

The bottom of a person's feet is the safest place to test for reactions to oils.

Children

As with any type of medication, keep all essential oils out of the reach of children. Do not use essential oils on or near children under 3 years old, unless supervised by a licensed healthcare practitioner. Do not use strong menthol oils, such as peppermint, on the necks or throats of children under 30 months old.

Pregnancy

Very few essential oils are completely safe for pregnant women throughout their entire pregnancies. Please be careful of being exposed to any scented products during your pregnancy and please be careful about exposing any pregnant women to scented products, especially pure essential oils, without their consent or foreknowledge. If you are pregnant, then please consult a licensed healthcare practitioner before using any essential oil or aromatic herb.

Diabetes

People with diabetes should always consult their physician prior to using any essential oil or aromatic herb, especially if they are taking insulin or other medications to control their diabetes.

Epilepsy

People with epilepsy need to avoid cajuput, clary sage, eucalyptus, fennel, hyssop, lavender (especially lavandula stoechas), rosemary, sage and thyme. They should consult a physician prior to using any other types of essential oils or aromatic herbs.

High Blood Pressure/Hypertension

People with high blood pressure need to avoid cajuput, cypress, eucalyptus, hyssop, rosemary, sage and thyme completely. They need to be cautious when using basil, birch, peppermint, tansy, tarragon and tansy. As should anyone with a medical condition, people with high blood pressure and/or hypertension should consult a physician prior to using any essential oils or aromatic herbs.

Hypotension

People with hypotension need to avoid clary sage and marjoram.

Liver Diseases

People with liver diseases need to avoid clove (bud and leaf), garlic, oregano, sassafras, thyme and vetiver.

There are numerous other contraindications for various health conditions. If you have any long-lasting or chronic health issues, consult a doctor prior to using essential oils. Other safety tips you should know are:

- **Never put oils directly into your eyes, nose or ears. Avoid rubbing your eyes or touching your contact lens if you have oil on your fingers. Some oils can damage contact lens, as well as highly irritate the eyes.**

- **Never put undiluted oil directly on the skin unless it is one of the few oils specifically labeled for such use.**

- **Never put undiluted essential oils directly in your bath water - always use some type of bath base to disperse the oils first.**

- Be aware that some essential oils can cause sensitivity to sunlight or intense lighting - be sure you check the label!

- Never store or use essential oils near electricity, open flames or sparks. Some of them are flammable and can catch on fire. If a fire does break out, use vegetable oil to put it out- water will just make it spread more, since essential oils are oil-soluble and not water-soluble.

- Never blindly follow someone else's recipe or formula - always ensure the recipe is adapted to your specific uniqueness.

- Never use essential oils to treat a specific ailment until you have completed a full assessment of the person being treated. This assessment must include mental, emotional, physical and spiritual health status, as well as environmental, genetic and past medical history factors.

- Always keep the phone number of a licensed healthcare practitioner handy in case of emergencies
- Always keep excellent records of which oils and scents you have experimented with and what your reactions have been. You will not regret doing this!

Most importantly of all safety tips is to remember that all scents can have an affect on you, as well as other people. Therefore, try to use any smell sparingly. Also, remember that in aromatherapy and the use of essential oils, more does not make a blend better. Always use essential oils very sparingly for all applications.

Chapter Nine: Where to Purchase and How to Store Essential Oils

Now that you have obtained a good foundation for your venture into aromatherapy, you are ready to purchase the essential oils for that venture. Purchasing the oils is a daring venture in its own right. Many online and off-line vendors sell essential oils and it is hard to know which ones to trust. Essential oils are produced all around the world and not every country does a good job of regulating the industry or setting trustworthy standards.

Therefore, I recommend that you stick to the better-established, reputable brands of essential oils. I also recommend that you go directly to the manufacturer to purchase the essential oils, whenever possible. Here is a list of the companies I recommend you check out (in alphabetical order):

- • doTerra - http://www.doterra.com/us/ - very potent essential oils, you may have to cut the amount used in recipes when using doTerra oils
- • Mountain Rose Herb - https://www.mountainroseherbs.com/
- • Native American Nutritionals- http://www.nativeamericannutritionals.com

• •   Young   Living   -
http://www.youngliving.com/en_US

There are numerous other companies that are reputable and worth checking out. To find some of these other companies, I suggest you visit the websites of professional associations for aromatherapists, such as The National Association for Holistic Aromatherapy (http://www.naha.org/)

Storing your Oils

Once you have purchased your essential oils and carrier oils, you will need to store them properly. Always keep the essential oils tightly closed, in a dark, cool area. Avoid light and use dark, blue or amber colored bottles to store essential oils. Exposure to air, light and heat can alter the chemical makeup and therapeutic benefits of essential oils. Moreover, most essential oils quickly evaporate when exposed to air.

You will also have to read the instructions for storage on the carrier oil's label carefully. Some of the oils will require refrigeration in between uses. Other carrier oils must be kept in dry areas and out of direct sunlight. If there are no instructions given on the label, you should be able to ask the manufacturer or a more-experienced aromatherapist.

Chapter Ten: Conclusion and Summary of Aromatherapy Principles to Remember

If you have taken the time to absorb the information provided in the first nine chapters, then you should now be ready to begin your hands-on venture into aromatherapy and essential oils. However, I do want to recap on some of the principles and debunked myths before I turn you lose to experiment with the recipes and blends I have provided for you in Part 2. These principles are:

1) Always choose scents and blends based on your own uniqueness. No two people are identical and therefore smells do not affect any two people in an identical manner. What works well for another person may be harmful to you. Let your own instincts guide you!

2) Be extremely cautious of over-exposure to all olfactory stimuli - remember that you are contributing to the constant bombardment of environmental smells just as much as anyone else is!

3) Learn to discern fact from fiction - be aware of the sales hype, myths and half-truths that abound in the media. Essential oils are not instant cure-alls to be randomly used for every occasion.

4) Always remember to do a skin test prior to using an essential oil and always add in just one drop at a time when blending oils. Take a whiff before proceeding to the next drop.

Please, never take your sense of smell for granted! The sense of smell is essential to survival. Over-exposure to various olfactory stimuli and chemicals can destroy this valuable asset. Your sense of smell affects your mental, emotional, spiritual and physical health every second that you are alive. So take responsibility for protecting your sense of smell and be aware of how you are affecting someone else's sense of smell too.

Moreover, remember that essential oils should be treated with the same cautionary awareness as any other type of medicine - they are very potent and are what most modern medicines are based on. Do not leave essential oils in the reach of children or pets! Just as you would not take prescribed medication without needing them, please do not use essential oils unless the need arises. Even in ancient times, essential oils were not used on a daily basis for pure pleasure.

Remember that no two people react to smells in an identical manner, whether the smell is pleasant or unpleasant. All reactions to scents are based on individual memories that have been associated with that smell, and what you consider pleasant and comforting, another person may find obnoxious and emotionally disturbing. Thus, all living creatures in interpreting non-verbal messages use the sense of smell. Be aware of the messages you are sending to other living creatures, as it does affect all your interpersonal relationships with those other creatures!

Please also remember not to fall for all the hype in the media and various marketing techniques. Take time to distinguish fact from fiction and think about the topics that have been briefly touched upon in the prior chapters. These are the myths that have been debunked:

- *Something is not safe to use just because it is "natural" or "organic" - some natural, organic things can be very toxic, including many of the essential oils.*
- *Not every essential oil or pleasant smell is used in traditional aromatherapy or is used to treat ailments.*
- *No two people react to smells in the same manner, so there is no such thing as a recipe, essential oil or blend of oils that is safe for every human being to use. Every essential oil comes with its own set of contraindications - pay close*

attention to those contraindications and your own level of sensitivity!

- *No two people will derive identical benefits from any identical scents - each person is a unique being and has unique reactions to every scent, each time he or she is exposed to that scent. Do not expect to receive the same benefits each time you use an essential oil. Do not expect to receive the same benefits that someone else received from using the same oils.*
- *It is not simply a matter of going out and buying a set of essential oils to cure all your ailments. There are over 700 essential oils and not all of them cure ailments. It takes years of practice and experimenting with essential oils to find which ones work best for you as a unique individual. In addition, it usually takes a blend of oils combined with other methods of alternative healing to treat any ailment sufficiently. Aromatherapy is more suited to allopathic treatments than for chronic, long-term illnesses.*

I think that about sums up all the primary concepts and myths. Now you can go have fun experimenting with the recipes in Part 2. Just remember to do the self-assessment prior to applying the treatments. Also remember to use some commonsense and adapt each of the formulas to match your own personal preferences.

Chapter Eleven: Measurements

Before you can mix your own blends or try out the recipes in this book, you will need to know how to measure the drops properly. When mixing the blends, please remember that using more drops of essential oils does not increase the therapeutic benefits of the overall blend. Here are the measurements you will need to know:

- 1 ml. = 30 drops
- 7.5 ml - 225 drops = 1/4 oz
- 10 ml. = 300 drops = 1/3 oz.
- 15 ml. = 450 drops = 1/2 oz.
- 30 ml. = 900 drops = 1 oz.
- 20 eye dropper drops = 30 bottle drops (blops)

When mixing blends for these applications, use:

- **Baths** - 8-12 drops in tub of water, 15-20 drops in soap base - never use neat oils in bath water

- **Body wraps** - 10-15 drops in spray bottle, mixed well with warm water

- **Compress/inhalation** - 4-6 drops in 1-2 pints warm water (usually a bowl of water)

- **Diffuser** - 15 -20 drops, neat - Do not use carrier oils or enfleurages (jasmine, gardenia, etc.) in a diffuser.

- **Douche** - 3-4 drops of tea tree oil per pint of water

- **Emulsifier** - 4 drops to 1 drop essential oil

- **Face oils, full-body oils and shower gels** - 15 drops in 1 oz. , 50-60 drops in 2 oz. of carrier oil

- **Facial mask** - 5 drops

- **Hair treatments** - 25 drops in 1 oz. jojoba oil

- **Massage oil** - 40-50 drops in 4 oz., typically should be 10 drops per 1 oz. of carrier oil

- **Meridians, pressure points and acute conditions** - 200-240 drops per 4 oz/ carrier oil
- **Ointment for specific area** - 40-50 drops in 2 oz. of carrier oil
- **Sore muscles** - 100-120 drops in 4 oz. of carrier oil

Please remember that oils are not water-soluble. Rinse them off with vegetable oil, hot soapy water or high-grade alcohol. Also, remember that some essential oils are flammable. If a fire breaks out, do not try to use water to put the fire out - use some type of vegetable oil or other carrier oil to extinguish it. Water will only help spread the flames, while the oil will help disperse the essential oil and keep the fire from spreading further

Chapter Twelve: Self- assessment

Prior to using any essential oil, it is important that you conduct a self-assessment. This self-evaluation should be carried out each time you utilize any products containing essential oils, even if you made the blend yourself. The types of questions you should be asking yourself are:

1) What is my musculo-skeletal health history? Think in terms of current and past physical health conditions, i.e. fibromyalgia, bone diseases, broken bones, lupus and any other physical type of ailment that may be influencing your body. Also, think about the type and frequency of any exercise you have had or are doing.

2) What is my circulatory health history? Think in terms of current and past aerobic activity, heart conditions, varicose veins, blood pressure ailments, blood clots, lymph-edema and anything else that may be affecting your circulatory system.

3) What is my respiratory health history? Think in terms of deep breathing exercises, breathing difficulties, sinus problems, allergies and anything else that may be affecting your respiratory system.

4) What is my skin's health history? Think in terms of special skin care regimes, hydrotherapy, allergies, rashes, athlete's foot, warts and contagious diseases.

5) What is my digestive system's health history? Are my nutritional habits excellent, average or poor? Think about any constipation, gas/bloating, diverticulitis, irritable bowel syndrome or any other digestive problems you may have had or are experiencing.

6) What is my reproductive system's health history? Am I pregnant? If so, what stage of pregnancy am I at? Also, think in terms of PMS, dysfunction and any other conditions that affect your reproductive system.

7) What is my nervous system's health history? Think in terms of current and past bouts of stress, fatigue, chronic fatigue syndrome, chronic pain, numbness/tingling, sleep disorders, herpes/shingles and any other factors that have or are affecting your nervous system.

8) What is my history with infectious diseases? Do I have AIDS, hepatitis, or any other types of infections diseases? Did I ever have any infectious diseases?

9) What type of other conditions do I have or have I had? Think in terms of cancer, diabetes, eating disorders, depression, drug addiction, alcohol addiction, nicotine addiction, caffeine addiction, desires for weight loss or weight gain and reshaping your body or health in some way.

10) What is my history of accidental injuries? Think in terms of vehicular accidents, work-related injuries, slips and falls, burns and anything else that may have caused you some type of conscious or subconscious trauma.

11) What is my mental/emotional health history? Think in terms of any specific disorders you have been diagnosed with are may think you have but have not sought out medical attention for. Think of A.D.D., dyslexia, grief, phobias, PTSD, OCD, generalized anxiety, mood changes, temper outbursts and any other intense emotions and mental conditions that might be affecting you or have affected you in the past.

12) What is my stress economy? Think in terms of levels of stress and what types of stress you are under at home, work and social events. Also, think about your attitude towards these stress factors, as well as what you are feeling today.

13) What are my energy, creative life force and sexual drive like? Am I hyperactive, fidgety or restless? Am I balanced, with a feeling of well-being? Am I uninspired, sluggish, tired and run down? What are my problematic areas?

14) What is spiritual health history? Think in terms of serenity levels of high, average and low. Do you feel grounded, centered, balanced and connected to others and your environment? Think about what spiritual disciplines you are practicing. Are you integrating your spiritual beliefs into your daily life routine? Are there any spiritual issues that may be affecting your health or that have affected it in the past?

15) What messages are my body, mind, heart and spirit trying to send each other? Am I paying attention to those messages? Are these ailments caused by an emotional, spiritual, mental, physical or combination of factors?

I know that this may seem like a long list of questions to go through each time you reach for an essential oil. However, once you get in the habit of living your life on a conscious level, then this type of assessment does not take very long to do. Moreover, doing the assessment each time provides you with much better results than otherwise. It may even save you the trouble of applying an essential oil treatment, simply by making you aware of what the real issue is. Most people tend to blame their physical health problems strictly on physical causes. This is because it is much easier to change physical activities than it is to change one's thoughts and emotions. Nevertheless, most physical pains are actually the result of the person's emotions and thoughts, and not due to physical strain or other physical factors. This is especially true of headaches, back pain and tense muscles.

Chapter Thirteen: Skin Care with Essential Oils

Skin makes up the largest portion (20%) of a person's body and is its largest organ. The skin's primary functions are to protect against microbes, infections and the elements. It aids in body temperature regulation and our sense of touch, especially when we are sensing pain or cold and heated objects. The outer layer, which is called the epidermis, is a waterproof barrier that creates the person's skin tone. The layer beneath the epidermis, which is called the dermis, consists of hair follicles, sweat glands and tough connective tissue. The deepest layer, which is called the hypodermis, consists of fat and connective tissue. When using essential oils, it is important to remember that some of the oils are absorbed through the skin while others are absorbed into the skin itself. Since the skin is so important to good health, I have included several recipes to aid you in protecting your skin's health. Please adapt the ingredients to suit your personal preferences and needs. You can refer to the lists of oils and their benefits and contraindications in Part 1 as you go about adapting these recipes and formulas.

Skin Care - Basic Instructions

Step 1: Activate the capillary circulation and open the pores by massaging your face and neck.

Step 2: Use a cleansing lotion, compress, facial steam bath or mask to clean the skin. Do not use a steam bath or mask if you have couperose, as these increase the circulation and may cause more capillaries to be broken.

Step 3: Use compresses made with cypress, juniper or bergamot to close the pores.

Step 4: Apply a moisturizing cream or oil (i.e. aloe vera gel with a few drops of essential oils added) to protect the skin.

Please note that facial lotions and creams may become unstable or rancid, so should be made up just prior to using it for skin care regimens. To make up the lotions and cream, pour some unscented carrier cream or lotion into your hand, add in three drops of essential oil and mix well with your fingertips. Then apply the mixture to your face.

Facial Compresses

Place five drops of the chosen blend of oils in a bowl of warm water. Soak cotton balls or a washcloth in the mixture then apply the cotton or cloth to your face for five minutes.

You may repeat this procedure up to three times in one session.

Facial masks

Cleansing, revitalizing and nourishing, masks aid in the elimination of dead cells and stimulate the local blood circulation. To make a mask, combine a few spoonfuls of clay or soaked oatmeal with a teaspoon of wheat germ oil in a bowl. Add in five drops of essential oil and stir the mixture. Then add in floral water or herbal tea. Use your fingertips and circular motions to apply the mixture to your face. Let it dry 10-15 minutes, and then use a wet washcloth to remove it gently. After you have removed the entire mask, apply floral water to your face to close the pores.

Facial Steam Baths

Place 5-10 drops of selected essential oils in a bowl of hot water and mix well. Use a large towel to cover your head as you bend forward over the bowl. Let the steam hit your face for 15 minutes. Make sure to keep your eyes closed or wear safety goggles that seal tightly around your eyes.

Body Wrap

Place a blanket on a comfortable, waterproofed horizontal surface. You can use plastic foil, a vinyl tablecloth or a plastic shower curtain to waterproof the surface. Place a large bath towel on top of the plastic covering. Next, combine 10-15 drops of the chosen blend of oils with 12 ounces of hot water in a spray bottle. Shake the spray bottle to ensure it is mixed well, and then spray the mixture on the towel. Make sure you constantly shake the bottle as you are spraying. After you have completely dampened the towel, lie on the towel and wrap yourself up with the towel, plastic covering and blanket. To make this even more relaxing, warm up the blanket and towel prior to wrapping your body in them.

Selection of Essential Oils for Skin Care

Some essential oils work better than others do when it comes to skin care. Just as you have to choose prefabricated products carefully, you also have to choose which essential oils best suit you personally. Here is a list of oils that are known to work best for each type of skin:

General Skin Care

- *Chamomile*
- *Lavender*

- *Carrot*
- *Geranium*
- *Lemon*
- *Ylang ylang*

Chapped Skin

- *Benzoin*
- *Chamomile*
- *Geranium*
- *Rose*
- *Sandalwood*

Dry Skin

- *Carrot*
- *Jasmine*
- *Peppermint*
- *Rosemary*
- *Clary sage*
- *Palmarosa*
- *Rose*
- *Sandalwood*

Inflamed Skin

- **Carrot**
- **Clary sage**
- **Geranium**
- **Lemon**
- **Patchouli**
- **Chamomile**
- **Floral water**
- **Lavender**
- **Myrrh**
- **Rose**

Normal Skin

- **Clary sage**
- **Lavender**
- **Geranium**
- **Ylang ylang**

Oily Skin

- **Basil**
- **Cedarwood**
- **Camphor**
- **Frankincense**

- *Geranium*
- *Lemon*
- *Lavender*
- *Ylang ylang*

Sensitive Skin

- *Chamomile(Roman)*
- *Melissa*
- *Rose*
- *Floral water*
- *Neroli*

Watery Skin/Water Retaining Skin

- *Grapefruit*
- *Lavender*
- *Rosemary*
- *Juniper*
- *Lemon*

For specific skin conditions:

Acne

- *Bergamot*
- *Eucalyptus*
- *Lavender*
- *Palmarosa*
- *Cajuput*
- *Juniper*
- *Niaouli*

Eczema

- *Chamomile*
- *Lavender*
- *Rose*
- *Cedarwood*
- *Patchouli*
- *Sage*

Rejuvenation

- *Benzoin*
- *Chamomile*
- *Carrot*
- *Frankincense*

- *Geranium*
- *Myrrh*

- *Lavender*
- *Rosemary*

Scars (keloid type)

Combine 20%-98% rose-hips oil seed with 1%-2% Helichrysum + 80% base oil

Seborrhea

- **Bergamot**
- **Lavender**

    Basil

- **Cypress**
- **Patchouli**

    Clary sage

Stretch Marks (prevention)

- **Cypress**

- **Neroli**

Sun photosynthesis (increases suntan)

Use bergamot to increase suntan, but avoid it if you do not want to become sunburned or over-sensitive to the sun.

- **Chamomile**

Wrinkles

- **Carrot**
- **Fennel**

- **Clary sage**
- **Frankincense**

- **Myrrh**
- **Palmarosa**
- **Chamomile**

- **Lemon**
- **Patchouli**
- **Geranium**

Bois-de-Rose

In most instances, it is best to use floral water instead of essential oils for skin care applications. It is milder and easier to use and do not irritate the skin as easily. You can also substitute floral water for water in most of the skin care recipes.

Sample Recipe:

As an example of how to combine a skin care blend for skin rejuvenation- Combine 1 drop of rosemary verbena, 1 drop spike lavender (10% camphor), 1 drop neroli with a carrier oil, lotion, gel or cream. For acne, use the same recipe and add in 1 drop of thyme linolol.

Chapter Fourteen: Hair Care with Essential Oils

Just as it is vital to care for your skin properly, it is essential to care for your hair properly. Contrary to popular belief, hair serves more of a purpose than just being an outward expression of self. Hair aids the skin with protection, regulation of body temperature and the evaporation of perspiration. It also acts as sense organs. The arrectores pilorum muscles (a bundle of smooth muscle fibers) are situated in the obtuse angle between the surface of skin and the root of a hair. These muscles respond to coldness and to emotions, creating goose pimples when they contract. Tugging the hair is sometimes used in reflexology treatments for the 100+ reflexology points located on a human's head. Since hair care is essential to good health, I have included the following recipes to aid you.

Instructions for Scalp Rub - Apply floral water using a Q-tip, or else combine ¼ oz. essential oil with 4 oz. grain alcohol or sweet almond oil, mix well and then apply to scalp using a Q-tip.

Instructions for shampoo or hair conditioner - Mix ¼ oz. essential oil in 16 oz. of your favorite type of unscented shampoo or conditioner. The following list provides you with some ideas of which essential oils work best, so choose any single oil or combination of oils that you prefer:

Dandruff

- **Cade**
- **Rosemary**
- **Thyme**
- **Eucalyptus**

- **Cedarwood**
- **Cypress**
- **Lavender**
- **Tea Tree**

Dry Hair

- **Cade**
- **Lavender**

- **Cedarwood**
- **Rosemary**

Hair Loss

- **Cedarwood**

- **Juniper**

- *Lavender*
- *Sage*
- *Rosemary*
- *Cypress*

Normal Hair

- *Chamomile*
- *Ylang Ylang*
- *Geranium*
- *Lavender*
- *Rosemary*
- *Lemon*

Oily Hair

- *Lemongrass*
- *Basil*
- *Rosemary*
- *Cypress*

Chapter Fifteen: Relaxation, Stimulation and Stress Relief via Baths and Massages

We each have our own natural cycles of energy. Unfortunately, those energy cycles do not always match our busy lifestyles. We may feel tired, sluggish and uninspired at a time when we need to be energetic, ambitious and alert. Sometimes we are feeling too energetic, anxious or stressed out to sleep soundly. With stress being associated with all the top sources of death around the globe, I think it is appropriate to include a chapter on ways to stimulate energy, as well as ways to relax and relieve stress.

The most beneficial methods to aid a person over all are baths and massages. Therefore, the following section gives recipes for bath salts, as well as bath and body lotions/oils. However, the following list just briefly touches upon some of the factors that can make a bath either restful and calming or relaxing while energizing you.

Baths

Baths can be calming or energizing, depending on these factors:

- Lighting - Use mildly bright or colored lights or natural sunlight to energize, use dim light or candle light for restful, calming bath or shower
- Scents - Use stimulating scents to energize, use calming or sedative aromas to calm down
- Temperature of water - The colder the water is, the more energizing it becomes (unless it reaches freezing temperatures, which can then cause hypothermia). Too hot of water may cause hyperthermia. To reduce fevers, take a bath in water that is equal to the room temperature. To lower your energy to a calm, restful state, take a warm or hot bath.
- Audio stimulants/relaxers - As with everything else in life, music comes with its own set of energy ranges. What one person finds stimulating, another person may find de-energizing, so experiment with music and see which is which for your own personal preferences. However, usually the faster the beat is, the more energizing the music may be. In addition, the higher the voice range, the more energizing it may be.
- External distractions - I.e. people interrupting bath, unpleasant background noises, unpleasant odors, messy or cluttered room
- Length of time in bath - Short, cold showers are more energizing than long, warm showers.

Instructions for Basic Bath Salt

Combine 3 cups salt (either Epsom or Dead Sea or Rock Salt) with 30-60 drops of your favorite essential oil in a large bowl (preferably ceramic or stainless steel, as plastic absorbs essential oils). Mix well. Then place in your storage jars. You may also add in ½ cup of baking soda, if you wish to use it as a water or skin softener.

If you want to add color to the salts, then use 5-15 drops of food coloring. You can also add in flowers, flower petals or dried leaves if you wish, although they can become irritating as they float around in the bath water.
These are the recommended oils for both, bath and massages:

Pain Relief

- **Eucalyptus**
- **Marjoram**
- **Rosemary**
- **Lavender**
- **Peppermint**

Energizing/Uplifting

- *Basil*
- *Bergamot*
- *Juniper berry*
- *Litsea cubeba*
- *Niaouli*
- *Ravensara*
- *Rosemary*
- *Spruce*

- *Bay (Laurel)*
- *Black pepper*
- *Lemon*
- *Marjoram (sweet)*
- *Pine*
- *Rose*
- *Spearmint*
- *Thyme*

Restful/Calming

- *Bergamot*
- *Cedarwood*

- *Chamomile (German and Roman)*
- *Clary sage*
- *Frankincense*
- *Geranium*
- *Lavender*
- *Mandarin*
- *Marjoram (sweet)*
- *Orange (sweet)*
- *Patchouli*
- *Rose*
- *Sandalwood*
- *Vetiver*
- *Ylang ylang*

Must remember that some of these essential oils will make you sensitive to sunlight or other forms of intense lighting (i.e. bergamot), so read the labels very carefully prior to using them.

Massages

Numerous styles of massages and massage strokes exist. The most well known style of full-body massage is called Swedish or Classic

Massage. The five primary strokes in Swedish massage are designed to both relax and stimulate the various body parts. Swedish massage techniques include:

Effleurage

Long, smooth sliding or gliding strokes, mostly used on the back, legs and arms- breaks up knots and tension in muscles

Petrissage

Kneading of muscles, typically used in smaller areas of the body for deeper tissue penetration

Friction

A vigorous rubbing motion that produces heat by friction - typically used to warm up the muscles in preparation for deeper tissue massages

Shaking/Vibration

Exactly what it sounds like! The technique is a slight rocking motion that is used to loosen and relax the muscles and shake the person's tension loose.

Tapoment

Light, rhythmic beating or tapping used to loosen, relax and energize muscles - typically done on end of massage session to help the person transit from a deep, relaxed state into a more energized, alert state

The massage therapist will use any combination of these five strokes either to relax the person or to energize the person, depending on the purpose of the massage. Shorter, more energizing styles of massage therapy include on-site seated massages, reflexology sessions, sports massages and Rolfing. Like Swedish massage sessions, energy-work types of massage sessions, such as shiatsu, polarity and reiki, tend to be more calming and restful.

Factors that influence the results obtained from massages are:

- **Lighting** - The dimmer the lighting is, the more calming and restful the massage is

- **Audio enhancers** - As with baths, the type of music or audio enhancers help to make the massage either restful or energizing

- **Type and duration of massage** - refer to previous paragraphs

- **Type of touch and person's comfort with being touched** - some types of touch are more energizing than other types (see aforementioned strokes) and each therapist has their own unique touch. Some can use feather-light touches and other therapists are very heavy-handed. In addition, some people have more of a trust issue than other people do and have difficulty relaxing around other people

- **External interference** - Noises, lighting, session interruptions, inconsistent or sudden cessation of touch or sound

- **Internal interference** - Health issues, inability to set aside mental or emotional issues

- **Scents** - Type of aromas used, person's unique response to smells

The same essential oils may be used in massage creams, lotions and oils as are used in bath salts and bath oils. However, to make sure it is easy to use for massages, I would recommend just buying the unscented Biotone massage gel, oil or lotion. I personally prefer gels to lotions and oils. This is because lotions tend to soak in too quickly during a massage and oils tend to leave the skin, especially the feet and hands, feeling oily and slippery after the massage is over. However, you can use any of your favorite carrier oils or any unscented body lotion that you prefer. Please refer back to Chapter Three, Skin Care with Essential Oils, to determine which oils are best for you to use in your bath, massage and body oil blends.

Chapter Sixteen- Essential Oils for Common Ailments and Well-being

As you can see from the following list, I mostly utilize just one blend of oils to treat numerous common ailments. This brings up the point that you do not have to use a wide variety of essential oils on a daily basis. You can choose a few essential oils that are the archetypes of their families and just dilute them down as needed to fit into specific applications. Here is a list of common ailments and conditions that can be addressed via essential oils:

Abdominal Cramping or Menstrual Pain

2 drops tangerine, 2 drops jasmine, 1 drop of clary sage, and 4 drops lavender mixed well with light carrier oil - I use 1 oz. of oil when utilizing this blend for baths

Arthritis

My aromatherapy mentor always recommended using equal parts (2%-5%) helichrysum (Aka Everlasting Immortelle) and eucalyptus citriodora in base oil. Mix well and apply to joints for immediate pain relief. I prefer just using lavender mixed with a bath base and taking a long soak in hot bath water when I am feeling stiff and sore.

Back Problems

Do self-assessment first- physical issues typically cause 2% of all back pain - most back pain is the result of emotional/mental issues. Lavender works well for all types of pain and can be used via massage oil, body lotion, creams, ointments, baths or diffusers.

Bruises

I use the same blend for bruises as I use for depression, headaches, stress relief and insomnia, which is the 2 drops tangerine, 2 drops jasmine, 1 drop clary sage, and 4 drops lavender mixed well with a light carrier oil

Cold and Flu

My favorite blend (2 drops tangerine, 2 drops jasmine, 1 drop clary sage, and 4 drops lavender mixed well with carrier oil) works well to relieve the aches and pains associated with colds and flues. However, I prefer long soaks in the tub for pain relief so I typically use 1 oz. of oil when utilizing this blend for baths, I also use Vitamin C citrus juices, chicken noodle soup, Echinacea capsules, eucalyptus or honey lemon cough drops, and herbal teas (green, white, Chamomile or any of the mint family). I think the best way to treat colds and flu is to get plenty of bed rest, drink many fluids and increase your Vitamin C intake.

Depression and Sadness

My favorite blend for depression/sadness consists of 2 drops tangerine, 2 drops jasmine, 1 drop clary sage, and 4 drops lavender mixed well with a light carrier oil - I use 1 oz. of oil when utilizing this blend for baths

Headaches

Same blend as for colds, flu, depression and stress relief

Pain Relief

My favorite way of relieving pain is via massages and baths. However, I do a self-assessment prior to attempting to relieve any pain, as the majority of all pain is due to emotional and mental causes rather than physical causes. I try to cope with those issues as best that I can. Then I use my favorite blend of 2 drops tangerine, 2 drops jasmine, 1 drop of clary sage, and 4 drops lavender mixed well with light carrier oil if doing a massage or I use 1 oz. of oil when utilizing this blend for baths.

Minor Skin Injuries

Combine 2 tbs. of grapeseed oil, olive oil or other carrier oil with 10 drops of lavender and 5 drops of tea tree or thyme. Mix well and apply to wound. Seek medical attention for deep wounds, heavily bleeding wounds, wounds caused by rusty objects and any wound that does not heal within a few days.

Stress Relief

2 drops tangerine, 2 drops jasmine, 1 drop clary sage, and 4 drops lavender mixed well with a light carrier oil - I use 1 oz. of oil when utilizing this blend for baths

The aforementioned favorite blend that I use happens to be good for numerous ailments. I like it because it can also be diffused in many ways, including massage gels and bath oils. This blend is good for:

- Anxiety

- Bronchitis

- Bruises

- Colds

- Depression

- Digestive system

- Energy
- Frigidity (good for people with trust and intimacy issues)
- Grief/emotional shock
- Headaches
- Infectious disease prevention
- Impotency
- Insomnia
- Insect repellant
- Menopause
- Menses and PMS
- Nervous tension
- Tension
- Respiratory system
- Sadness
- Stress
- Water retention

The main reason most of these benefits can be derived from this blend (2 drops tangerine, 2 drops of jasmine, 1 drop of clary sage, and 4 drops of lavender) is that the blend contains lavender. Lavender is frequently touted as the universal essential oil due to its numerous therapeutic benefits. Between using lavender, eucalyptus and tea tree oils, you can obtain just about any of the therapeutic benefits that essential oils provide humans. Therefore, if you are able to, start out by exploring how these three oils can fit into your life. Nevertheless, remember to use all essential oils sparingly.

Chapter Seventeen - Essential Oil for Home

Just as lavender is great for beauty and various ailment treatments, it is also an excellent choice for enhancing the home and natural cleaning products. Cinnamon, lemon, pine and peppermint also work well in homemade cleaning products. Some other choices for suitable essential oils are citronella, citrus oils (i.e. lime and sweet orange), eucalyptus, lemongrass, rosemary, tea tree and thyme. The best choice depends on what type of surface you are cleaning, as well as which type of benefits you wish to derive from adding essential oils to the cleaning solution. Here are sample recipes for various homemade cleaning products:

Air Fresheners

To freshen a room, mix a few drops of any of the aforementioned oils with water in a spray bottle. Shake well and then spray a mist into the area you wish to refresh. You can also just add the essential oils directly onto cotton balls and place the cotton balls around the room. This cotton ball method also works to get odors out of the refrigerator. Another method to absorb odors is to place an absorbent material, such as baking soda, cat litter or a slice of bread, in a small opened container in an out-of-the way area of the room and just leave it there until the odors have been absorbed.

Carpet Deodorizer/ Shampoo

To deodorize a carpet, combine a few drops of lime oil with baking soda and let it set long enough for the baking soda to absorb the essential oils. Then sprinkle the mixture over the carpet and let it set for around 15-20 minutes. Afterward, vacuum the carpet. To shampoo the carpet, thoroughly mix 10-15 drops of lemon oil with one gallon of carpet cleaning solution. This helps to pull out stains while deodorizing the carpet.

Another method of shampooing the carpet is to mix well 10 drops of peppermint oil, 3 cups of water and ¾ cup of liquid castile soap in a blender to create foam. Use a damp sponge to rub the foam into soiled areas and then let it dry completely. Once it is thoroughly dried, simply vacuum the carpet.

General Purpose Disinfectant

Thoroughly mix 8-10 drops of thyme, 2 cups of hot water and ¼ cup of washing soda in a spray bottle. Spray the solution on the surface

and then wipe surface off with a damp sponge
or cloth.

Handy Wipes

Make up some cotton cleaning cloths, cutting
the cloth to match the size of the storage
container. Old t-shirts are great for this
purpose! Next, fill the container with a
thoroughly mixed mixture of 6-8 drops of
essential oils, 1 oz. of liquid castile soap and 1
cup of water. Use the cloths as needed to wipe
up any spills, then simply wash the cloths and
return them to their storage container in
between uses. Make sure you keep the
container tightly closed in between uses so the
essential oils will not evaporate.

Liquid Dishwasher Detergent

Fill a 22 oz. squirt bottle with liquid castile
soap (dilute the soap as directed if it is
concentrated), then mix in a combination of
15- 20 drops lime oil, 8-10 drops sweet orange
oil and 3-5 drops citrus seed extract. Just
wash the dishes as usual after adding 1-2
tbsp. of this mixture to the dishwasher.

Oven Cleaner

Remove the oven racks, set the oven
temperature to 250 degrees and preheat the

oven for 15 minutes. Next, let the oven cool down with the door open while you combine ½-cup salt, ¼ washing soda and 16 oz. of baking soda with just enough water to make a paste. After the oven has cooled downed enough to avoid being burned, yet is still warm, spread the paste on the oven's walls with a sponge or cloth. Let the paste set for 20-30 minutes, while you thoroughly mix up mixture of 8-10 drops of thyme, 8-10 drops of lemon with ¾ cup of white vinegar in a spray bottle. Once the paste has set for long enough, spray the walls with the vinegar/essential oil mixture and wipe the walls off. Be sure you completely rinse the walls off afterward. You can add more salt if you need more scrubbing power, as well as use steel wool to help scrub the tougher stains.

Toilet Antibacterial Cleanser

Thoroughly mix ¼ cup of liquid castile soap, 1 tbsp. of tea tree oil, 8-10 drops of eucalyptus oil (can substitute peppermint oil) with 2 cups of water in a spray bottle. Spray toilet surfaces with mixture and wipe off with a damp sponge or cloth.

Although the essential oils do add extra benefits, it is not necessary to over-expose you and your loved ones to these olfactory stimuli. You can make unscented natural homemade cleaning products from various combinations and single applications of:

- Baking soda (aka bicarbonate of soda)

- Citrus seed extract (frequently sold as grapeseed extract

- Lemon juice

- Liquid Castile soap (can also use the bar form of castile soap)

- Salt (kosher salt works best, but regular table salt works well too)

- Vinegar (white vinegar tends to work best in some applications, while apple cider vinegar works best in other applications)

- Washing soda (aka soda ash and sodium carbonate)

The most important thing to remember when using any type of cleaning product is to test the product out in an inconspicuous location prior to using it widespread on any surface. Some products may cause damage, such as fading, bleaching or structural damage to particular types of materials and surfaces. This is especially true for furniture fabrics, carpets, rugs and wood products.

Chapter Eighteen: Blends to Start your Journey to the World of Essential Oils

Health Care

Cold & flu Treatment

- Lavender essential oil   - 7 drops

- Myrtle essential oil - 5 drops

- Frankincense essential oil - 6 drops

- Eucalyptus essential oil - 2 drops

- Rosemary essential oil - 1 drop

Mix the oils together & massage on the soles of your feet hands and chest.

Stuffy Nose Treatment

- Tea tree essential oil - 3 drops

- Helichrysum essential oil - 1 drop

- Clove essential oil - 2 drops

- Eucalyptus essential oil - 3 drops

Mix them and apply under the nostrils or to the chest or spine.

Stuffy Nose Steam Inhalation Blend

- Eucalyptus essential oil - 6 drops
- Neroli essential oil – 4 drops
- Lemon essential oil - 3 drops

Add all 3 oils in 180ml distilled water in to a pan & heat. And cover your head with a towel. Remove the pan from the heat & allow the stream to be inhaled for 5 minutes.

Stuffy Nose Diffuser Blend

- Peppermint essential oil - 5 drops
- Lavender essential oil - 4 drops
- Eucalyptus essential oil - 4 drops
- Orange essential oil - 2 drops

Add all the in gradients in the diffuser and turn on the diffuser.

Stuffy Nose Bath Blend - 1

- Peppermint essential oil - 5 drops
- Rosemary essential oil - 4 drops
- Eucalyptus essential oil - 3 drops
- Tea tree oil - 2 table spoon

Mix all the essential oils in a small bowl and then pour into the warm bath water.

Stuffy Nose Bath Blend - 2

- Eucalyptus essential oil - 15 drops
- Helichrysum essential oil - 4 drops
- Clove essential oil - 6 drops

Mix all the ingredients in a small bowl. Add the oils to the warm water.

Stress Relief

Stress Relief Blend

- Jojoba oil - 30 ml
- Lavender oil - 8 drops

Mix the Lavender essential oil to Jojoba carrier oil and shake well. Use it as a diffuser or spray in your room. It is a stress buster and very effective.

Stress Relief Diffuser Blends

Blend 1

- Clary sage essential oil - 12 drops
- Orange essential oil - 4 drops
- Lavender essential oil - 4 drops

Blend 2

- Roman Chamomile essential oil- 8 drops
- Lavender essential oil - 8 drops

- Vetiver essential oil - 1 drop

Blend 3
- Bergamot essential oil - 12 drops
- Geranium essential oil - 4 drops
- Frankincense essential oil - 4 drops

Blend 4
- Chamomile essential oil - 8 drops
- German Chamomile essential oil - 2 drops
- Rose essential oil - 2 drops
- Geranium essential oil - 2 drops

Combine the oils in the well of the diffuser. Light the candle in the tea light diffuser or plug in the electric diffuser.

Stress Relief Massage Blends

Blend 1

- Geranium - 2 drops

- Frankincense- 2 drops

- Spruce - 1 drop

- Almond oil - 2 drops

- Patchouli - 1 drop

- Ginger - 1 drop

- Sage - 1 drop

Combine the essential oils in the 60 ml Almond carrier oil and stir thoroughly. Massage on the skin with medium pressure.

Blend 2

- Lavender essential oil -10 drops

- Chamomile essential oil - 6 drops

- Ylang. Ylang essential oil - 4 drops

- Sandalwood essential oil - 2 drops

- Carrier oil of choice - 60 ml

Add the essential oils in the carrier oil and stir thoroughly. Massage on the skin using medium pressure.

Blend 3
- Patchouli Essential oil - 4 drops
- Frankincense essential oil - 3 drops
- Bergamot essential oil - 3 drops
- Carrier oil of your choice - 60 ml

Add the essential oils in the carrier oil and stir to combine. Massage the recipe on the skin using medium pressure.

Skin Care

General Skin Care by Age

Blend 1 - Skin Care in 20s

- Chamomile - 5 drops

- Carrot - 1 drop

- Geranium - 8 drops

- Lavender - 5 drops

- Lemon - 3 drops

- Ylang Ylang - 8 drops

Mix all the oils in one tbsp. of floral water and massage your skin lightly twice a day.

Blend 2 - Skin Care in 30s

- Bergamot - 5 drops

- Lavender - 5 drops

- Palmarosa – 5 drops

- Clary sage - 5 drops

- Rose - 5 drops

- Patchouli - 1 drop

Mix all the oils in one tbsp. of floral water and massage your skin lightly twice a day.

Blend 3 - Skin Care in 40s

- Lavender - 10 drops

- Lemon - 8 drops

- Ylang Ylang - 7 drops

- Chamomile - 5 drops

Mix all the oils with one tbsp. of floral water and massage your skin lightly twice a day.

Blend 4 - Skin Care in 50s

- Lavender - 4 drops

- Carrot - 2 drops

- Geranium - 6 drops

Mix all the oils with one tbsp. of floral water and massage your skin lightly twice a day.

Chapped Skin Care Blends

Blend 1

- Benzoin - 2 drop
- Chamomile - 8 drops
- Geranium - 8 drops
- Rose - 10 drops
- Sandalwood - 2 drops

Mixed all oils with 2 tbsp Almond or Hazelnut or Apricot kernel oil and massage.

Blend 2

- Lavender - 10 drops
- Chamomile - 8 drops
- Geranium - 7 drops
- Sandalwood - 5 drops

Mix all the oils with one tbsp. of floral water and massage your skin lightly twice a day.

Blend 3

- Bergamot - 10 drops
- Chamomile - 8 drops
- Geranium - 7 drops
- Rose - 5 drops
- Patchouli - 3 drops
- Benzoin - 2 drops

Mix all the oils with one tbsp. of floral water and massage your skin lightly twice a day.

Inflamed Skin Blends

Blend 1

- Lavender - 10 drops
- Lemon - 5 drops
- Clary sage - 7 drops
- Myrrh - 5 drops
- Chamomile - 5 drops

Mix all oil with 30 ml of floral water and massage your skin lightly twice a day.

Blend 2

- Lavender - 10 drops
- Rose - 8 drops
- Geranium - 7 drops
- Clary sage - 5 drops
- Patchouli - 5 drops

Mix all the oils with 30 ml of floral water and massage your skin lightly twice a day.

Dry Skin Blends

Blend 1

- Peppermint - 5 drops

- Rose - 8 drops

- Rosemary - 7 drops

- Palmarosa - 7 drops

- Sandalwood - 3 drops

Mix all the oils with one tbsp. of floral water and massage your skin lightly twice a day.

Blend 2

- Lavender - 10 drops

- Clary sage - 8 drops

- Jasmine - 7 drops

- Rosemary - 7 drops

- Carrot - 3 drops

Mix all the oils with one tbsp. of floral water and massage your skin lightly twice a day.

Normal Skin Blends

Blend 1

- Lavender - 10 drops

- Geranium - 8 drops

- Ylang Ylang 5 drops

- Clary sage - 7 drops

- Patchouli - 5 drops

Mix all the oils with one tbsp. of floral water and massage your skin lightly twice a day.

Blend 2

- Tangerine - 5 drops

- Jasmine - 7 drops

- Clary sage - 2 drops

- Sandal wood - 3 drops

Mix all the oils with 1/2 tbsp. of floral water and massage your skin lightly twice a day.

Oily Skin Blends

Blend 1

- Basil - 10 drops

- Geranium - 7 drops

- Lavender - 8 drops

- Ylang Ylang - 5 drops

- Frankincense - 5 drops

Mix all the oils with one tbsp. of floral water and massage your skin lightly twice a day.

Blend 2

- Petitgrain - 5 drops

- Lemon - 5 drops

- Juniper - 10 drops

- Marjoram - 5 drops

- Cedarwood - 5 drops

Mix all the oils with one tbsp. of floral water and massage your skin lightly twice a day.

Sensitive Skin Blends

Blend 1

- Lavender - 10 drops
- Chamomile (Roman) - 8 drops
- Neroli - 7 drops
- Rose - 5 drops
- Sandalwood - 3 drops
- Patchouli 2 drops

Mix all the oils with one tbsp. of floral water and massage your skin lightly twice a day.

Blend

- Grapeseed oil - 8 drops
- Geranium - 7 drops
- Lavender - 5 drops
- Neroli - 5 drops
- Sandalwood - 5 drops

Mix all the oils with one tbsp. of floral water and massage your skin lightly twice a day.

Watery Skin/Water Sustaining Skin Blends

Blend 1

- Grapefruit 5 drop
- Lemon - 5 drops
- Lavender - 8 drops
- Rosemary - 7 drops
- Juniper - 5 drops
- Sandalwood - 5 drops

Mix all the oils with one tbsp. of floral water or Apricot kernel oil and massage your skin lightly twice a day.

Blend 2

- Petitgrain - 3 drops
- Bergamot 2 drops
- Lavender - 5 drops
- Rosemary - 5 drops
- Patchouli - 5 drops

Mix all the oils with one tbsp. of floral water or Apricot kernel oil and massage your skin lightly twice a day.

For Specific conditions
Acne Blends
Blend 1
- Bergamot - 3 drops

- Eucalyptus 2 drops

- Lavender - 8 drops

- Neroli - 7 drops

- Palmarosa - 5 drops

- Myrrh - 5 drops

- Base oil - Evening primrose or Almond

  oil 2 tbsp

Mix all the oils with two tbsp. of base oil (Evening primrose or Almond oil) and massage slowly on Acne after washing the affected area.

Blend 2
- Lavender - 10 drops

- Neroli - 5 drops

- Cajuput - 5 drops

- Chamomile - 5 drops

- Juniper - 5 drops

Mix all the oils with two tbsp. of base oil (Evening primrose or Almond oil) and massage slowly on Acne after washing the affected area.

Eczema Blends

Blend 1

- Lavender - 10 drops
- Chamomile - 8 drops
- Rose - 7 drops
- Clary sage - 5 drops
- Cedarwood - 5 drops
- Base Oil - Jojoba oil or Sesame oil

Mix all the oils with two tbsp. of base oil (Jojoba oil or Sesame oil) and massage slowly on the affected area after washing it.

Blend 2

- Lavender - 10 drops
- Clary sage - 7 drops
- Rosemary - 8 drops
- Neroli - 5 drops

- Patchouli - 5 drops

Mix all the oils with two tbsp. of base oil (Jojoba oil or Sesame oil) and massage slowly on the affected area after washing it.

Rejuvenation Blends

Blend 1

- Lavender - 15 drops
- Chamomile - 5 drops
- Geranium - 7 drops
- Rosemary - 8 drops
- Myrrh - 3 drops
- Frankincense - 2 drops
- Base Oil - Evening Primrose

Mix all the oils with two tbsp. of base oil (Evening Primrose) and massage slowly.

Blend 2

- Lavender - 10 drops
- Carrot - 5 drops
- Rosemary - 8 drops
- Chamomile - 7 drops
- Benzoin - 5 drops

Mix all the oils with two tbsp. of base oil (Evening Primrose) and massage slowly.

Seborrhea

Blend 1

- Bergamot - 6 drops
- Cypress – 3 drops
- Lavender 9 drops
- Patchouli - 3 drops
-    Base oil - Almond oil

Mix all the oils with 30 ml of base oil (Almond oil) and massage slowly.

Blend 2

- Basil 10 drops
- Clary sage - 8 drops
- Neroli - 5 drops
- Palmarosa - 7 drops
- Patchouli - 5 drops

Mix all the oils with 30 ml of base oil (Almond oil) and massage slowly.

Wrinkles Treatment by Age

Base Oil - Hazel nut or Sweet Almond oil

Skin Care in 20 s

- Lavender - 6 drops

- Neroli - 8 drops

- Palmarosa - 7 drops

- Fennel – 3 drops

- Myrrh - 3 drops

Mix all the oils with one tbsp of base oil (Hazel nut or Sweet Almond oil) and massage wrinkles twice a day

Skin Care in 30 s

- Lemon - 5 drops

- Yarrow - 5 drops

- Clary sage - 8 drops

- Carrot - 7 drops

- Patchouli - 3 drops

- Frankincense - 2 drops

Mix all the oils with one tbsp of base oil (Hazel nut or Sweet Almond oil) and massage wrinkles twice a day

Skin Care in 40 s

- Lavender - 10 drops
- Neroli - 8 drops
- Chamomile - 5 drops
- Geranium - 7 drops
- Patchouli - 3 drops
- Myrrh - 2 drops

Mix all the oils with one tbsp of base oil (Hazel nut or Sweet Almond oil) and massage wrinkles twice a day

Skin Care in 50 s

- Bois –de rose - 10 drops
- Rose - 8 drops
- Carrot - 7 drops

- Geranium - 5 drops

- Myrrh - 3 drops

- Frankincense - 2 drops

Mix all the oils with one tbsp of base oil (Hazel nut or Sweet Almond oil) and massage wrinkles twice a day

Hair Care
Eucalyptus Anti Dandruff Shampoo

- Cedar wood oil - 5 drops

- Grape seed oil - 10 drops

- Eucalyptus oil - 15 drops

- Mild shampoo - 60 ml

- Water - 60 ml

Mix all ingredients and heat until mixture is thick & even and set aside to cool. Use this as antidandruff shampoo.

Lavender Scalp Treatment

- Olive oil - 1 cup

- Lavender oil - 15 drops

- Egg yolk - 1 piece

Warm Olive oil for 5 minutes. After cooling the Olive oil mix 15 drops Lavender oil in it & shake. After that mix egg yolk and stir. Apply this mixture on hair and scalp. Wrap the head for 15 minutes then wash.

Lavender & Cedarwood Dandruff Blend

- Cedarwood oil - 2 drops
- Lavender oil - 2 drops
- Patchouli oil - 1 drop
- Tea tree oil - 2 tbsp.

Mix the oil together and stir thoroughly and massage the scalp and hair.

Dandruff Treatment with Tea tree

- Regular shampoo - 240 ml
- Tea tree oil - 10 drops

Mix tea tree oil with regular shampoo well and apply shampoo to wet hair and let the shampoo in your hair for 5 minutes. Rinse off the shampoo with cool water.

Dry Hair Care Blends

Peppermint Shampoo for Dry hair

- Spring water - 210 ml

- Liquid soap castile - 30 ml

- Peppermint oil - 2 tbsp

Boil spring water on a pot with soap castile and stir until fully boiled. Add peppermint oil and stir for 3 minutes. Remove the pot from fire and pour mixture into a glass bottle cover tightly and use this shampoo to the hair.

Sandalwood Conditioning Treatment

- Castor oil - 10 drops

- Jojoba oil - 10 drops

- Sandalwood oil 20 drops

- Egg yolk - 1 piece

Mix all ingredients in a pan on a low heat & stir the mixture until consistency in thick. Remove from heat and allow the mixture to cool. Apply as conditioner to the hair and leave it for 20 minutes. Rinse hair thoroughly.

Dry Hair Treatment with Lavender and Rosemary

- Lavender oil - 3 drops
- Rosemary oil - 2 drops
- Sandalwood oil - 2 drops
- Geranium oil - 1 drop
- Carrier oil - 2 tbsp.

Mix all oils in a small bowl thoroughly and rub it through your hair. Rinse with warm water.

Dry Hair Treatment with Cedarwood and Sandalwood

- Cedarwood oil - 2 drops
- Sandalwood oil - 5 drops
- Carrier oil - 1 tbsp.

Mix all oils into a small bowl thoroughly and rub it through your hair. Rinse with normal water.

Oily Hair Care Blends
Oily Hair Care with Lemon

- Soap stew - 4 ounces

- Rosemary - 3 drops

- Basil - 1 drop

- Lemon - 15 drops

- Cypress - 2 drops

Mix all the ingredients well in a blender and shake before use.

Blend for Shiny Hairs

- Soap stew - 4 ounces

- Thyme - 6 drops

- Eucalyptus - 7 drops

- Lavender - 3 drops

- Rosemary - 4 drops

Mix together well, shake before use.

Oily Hair Care with Basil shampoo

- Liquid castile soap - 4 ounces
- Vegetable glycerin - ½ tsp.
- Vitamin E - ¼ tsp.
- Aloe vera - 30 ml
- Basil oil - 5 drops

Mix all the ingredients and pour mix into a glass bottle and cover it tightly. Level properly and store. Use this as hair shampoo.

Oily Hair Care with Lavender and Rosemary

- Lavender oil - 1 drop
- Rosemary oil - 2 drops
- Lemon oil - 1 drop
- Peppermint oil -1 drop
- Cypress oil - 2 drop
- Carrier oil of choice - 2 tbsp

Shampoo your hair with your desired shampoo. Mix all the essential oil in a bowl and rub through your hair for 5 minutes rinse with warm water.

Hair Loss Treatment

Hair Loss Treatment with Rosemary & Jojoba

- Cypress oil - 2 drops
- Lavender oil - 1 drop
- Rosemary oil - 2 drop
- Jojoba oil - 2 tbsp.

Mix all the essential oil together in a small bowl then add the jojoba and stir massage the oils into your scalp and hair for about 5 minutes then rinse with warm water.

Hair Loss Treatment with Thyme and Jojoba

- Ylang ylang oil - 2 drops
- Cedarwood oil - 2 drops
- Thyme oil - 2 drops
- Geranium oil - 1 drop
- Jojoba oil - 2 tbsp

Add all oil into jojoba oil and stir thoroughly. Wash your hair with your choice of shampoo and then massage the essential. oil into your scalp. Leave it for 10 min. then rinse with warm water.

Normal Hair Care

Hair care with Lemon

- Soap stew - 4 ounces

- Geranium - 3 drops

- Carrot - 4 drops

- Lemon - 2 drops

- Borage - 4 drops

Mix all oils into soap stew properly and use it as shampoo.

Conditioning with Carrot and Geranium

- Lecithin base - 1 tbsp.

- Almond oil - 1 tbsp

- Peach kernel oil - 2 tsp.

- Carrot - 3 drops

- Geranium - 2 drops

Mix properly and apply all over the hair and leave for at least ten minutes before rinsing off.

Chamomile Shampoo

- Hot water - 1 and 1/2 cup
- Chamomile - 20 drops
- Chopped soap - 1 cup
- Glycerin - 1 tbsp.

Place hot water in bowl and add chamomile oil in it. Set the mix. For 15 minutes. Then add chopped soap in this mix. Let the mix stand for 3 min. then add glycerin in it & blend.

Pour the mixture into glass bottle. Use this to shampoo the hair.

Rose conditioning treatment

- Egg yolk - 1 piece
- Eucalyptus oil - 3 tsp.
- Lemon - 1 squeezed
- Cedar wood oil - 10 drops
- Rose oil - 15 drops

Mix all ingredient into a bowl. Apply mixture to the hair and leave it for 5 minutes. Rinse the hair thoroughly and dry.

Pain Relief

Pain Relief Blend

- Wintergreen essential oil - 4 drops
- Jojoba oil - 30 ml

Mix the oils in a glass or plastic bottle and shake well before use massage 3 drops on the painful area or diffuser in the room.

Chronic Pain Diffuser Blend with Basil and Valerian

- Basil essential oil - 6 drops
- Valerian essential oil - 6 drops
- Winter green essential oil - 2 drops

Combine all the ingredients & turn on the diffuser.

Chronic Pain Massage Blend

- Lavender essential oil - 6 drops

- Spruce essential oil - 4 drops

- Clove essential oil - 4 drops

- Carrier oil of choice - 60 ml

Add the essential oils into the carrier oil and stir. Apply the massage oil to the painful area with light pressure.

Joint Pain Diffuser Blend

- Roman Chamomiles essential oil - 6 drops

- Neroli essential oil - 3 drops

- Spruce essential oil - 3 drops

- Grapefruit essential oil - 2 drops

Add all the ingredients into the diffuser and turn it on.

Chronic pain diffuser Blend with Basil and Lavender

- Basil oil - 6 drops
- Lavender oil - 4 drops
- Winter green oil - 2 drops

Combine all ingredients and turn on the diffuser.

Chronic Pain Diffuser Blend with Fir needle & Nutmeg

- Fir needle - 4 drops
- Marjoram oil - 2 drops
- Nutmeg oil - 4 drops
- Rosemary oil - 2 drops

Combine all ingredients in the diffuser and turn on.

Chronic Pain Massage Blend

- Lavender oil - 6 drops

- Spruce oil - 4 drops
- Clove oil - 4 drops
- Carrier oil - 60 ml (of your choice)

Add essential oil into the carrier oil to apply the massage oil to the painful area with light pressure.

Pain Massage Blend with Peppermint & Rosemary

- Eucalyptus oil - 4 drops
- Lavender oil - 3 drops
- Rosemary oil - 3 drops
- Peppermint oil - 2 drops
- Marjoram oil - 3 drops

Mix all essential oil into carrier oil (60 ml) of your choice and massage gently.

Energizing/ Uplifting

Diffuser Blend with Basil & Rosemary

- Basil oil - 8 drops

- Rosemary oil - 6 drops

- Lemon oil - 6 drops

- Marjoram oil - 2 drops

Add all the ingredients into the diffuser and turn it on.

Energy Diffuser Blend with Bergamot & Spearmint.

- Bergamot - 5 drops

- Spearmint - 4 drops

- Neroli - 4 drops

- Bay (Laurel) – 2 drops

Mix all the ingredients in the diffuser & turn it on.

Energy Massage Blend with Basil & Rose

- Rose oil - 3 drops

- Lavender oil - 3 drops
- Basil oil - 3 drops
- Spearmint - 2 drops
- Bergamot – 2 drops
- Carrier oil of choice 4 tbsp.

Combine all the essential oils in the carrier oil and stir. Massage with medium pressure.

Energy Boosting Massage Blend with Lemon & Peppermint

- Lemon - 5 drops
- Tangerine - 5 drops
- Peppermint - 3 drops
- Thyme - 5 drops
- Carrier oil of your choice - 60 ml

Combine the essential oils in the carrier oil and massage with medium pressure.

Lighting & Removing Older Scar

Blend 1

- Jasmine - 9 drops

- Geranium - 9 drops

- Patchouli - 3 drops

- Rosewood - 9 drops

Mix all oils and apply on the scar twice a day. And apply on older scar thrice a day. These essential oil will help with overall skin moisturizing & health.

Blend 2

- Lavender - 10 drops

- Helichrysum - 3 drops

- Sage - 8 drops

- Neroli - 7 drops

- Rosehip seed - 5 drops

- Hazelnut oil - 10 drops

Mix all oils and apply on the scar twice a day. And apply on older scar thrice a day. These essential oil will help with overall skin moisturizing & health.

Beauty & Bath Oils

For Radiant Skin

Normal Skin Blend

- Lavender 12 drops
- Neroli - 5 drops
- Palmarosa 10 drops
- Frankincense - 3 drops

Dry Skin Blend

- Palmarosa - 10 drops
- Chamomile German - 8 drops
- Carrot - 5 drops
- Bois de rose - 7 drops

Greasy Skin Blend

- Lavender - 15 drops
- Cypress - 10 drops
- Ylang Ylang - 5 drops

Mix the oils well and use it.

Insomnia

General Insomnia Blend

- Clary sage - 3 drops
- Vertiver - 2 drops
- Varian - 1 drop
- Lavender - 2 drops

Use 3 drops per bath or a 2 drops in 1 tsp. vegetable oil for a body rub.

Foot Bath Blend

- Lavender - 2 drops
- Chamomile Roman - 6 drops
- Marjoram - 6 drops
- Valerian - 2 drops

Use 2 drops in a foot bath.

Gastric Flatulence

Blend 1

- Cardamom - 2 drops

- Peppermint - 3 drops
- Vegetable oil - 1 tsp

Mix all the oils and rub over the whole of the abdomen in a clockwise direction.

Blend 2
- Spearmint - 3 drops
- Coriander - 2 drops
- Vegetable oil - 1 tsp

Mix all the oils and rub over the whole of the abdomen in a clockwise direction.

Constipation

Massage in a clock wise direction over the stomach as deeply as you can without causing discomfort, then over the lips and lower back. Do this three times a day.

Constipation Blends

Blend 1

- Black pepper - 5 drops
- Cardamom - 5 drops
- Patchouli 15 drops
- Vegetable oil 1 tbsp

Mix all the oils and apply as mentioned before

Blend 2

- Fennel - 5 drops
- Ginger - 5 drops
- Sandalwood - 15 drops
- Vegetable oil - 1 tbsp

Mix all the oils and apply as mentioned before

Blends for Home

Air Fresheners Blends

Blend 1

- Orange - 10 drops

- Chamomile - 10 drops

- Lemon - 8 drops

- Rose - 5 drops

- Distilled water 180 ml.

Mix all ingredients in the spray bottle and shake the bottle to combine. Spray the desired room with the air freshener.

Blend 2

- Bergamot - 10 drops

- Sandalwood oil - 10 drops

- Clove oil - 5 drops

- Ylang Ylang oil - 5 drops

Combine the essential oils in the diffuser and turn it on.

Blend 3 for Summers

- Lemon - 10 drops

- Geranium 4 drops

- Pent grain - 3 drops

- Sandalwood - 3 drops

  Combine the essential oils in the diffuser and turn it on.

Blend 4 for Autumn/Winter

- Orange - 8 drops

- Frankincense - 3 drops

- Benzoin - 2 drops

- Geranium - 7 drops.

  Combine the essential oils in the diffuser and turn it on.

Cleaner/ Disinfectant

Lemon Disinfecting Cleaner

- Lemon - 15 drops
- Eucalyptus - 5 drops
- Distilled water - 180 ml.

Combine all ingredients in the spray bottle and shake thoroughly before use.

Tea Tree Disinfecting cleaner

- Tea tree oil - 10 drops
- Lemon oil - 5 drops
- Distilled water - 60 ml
- Sea salt - ½ tsp

Combine all the ingredients in the spray bottle and shake before use. A new batch of the cleaner should be made each time it in needed.

Kitchen Fresheners
Air Spray for Kitchen

- Rosemary - 10 drops
- Lavender - 10 drops
- Lemon - 5 drops
- Lime - 3 drops
- Eucalyptus - 2 drops
- Distilled water 120 ml.

Mix all oils in distilled water into a spray bottle and shake before use.

Cleaning Kitchen Blend

- Lemon - 10 drops
- Lavender - 8 drops
- Eucalyptus - 5 drops
- Bois de rose - 8 drops
- Palmarosa - 3 drops

Mix all oils in 120 ml of water and use this blend to wipe the kitchen surfaces including the floor. This blend can be used as disinfecting and had antibacterial property

Essential Oils for Clothes

Essential oils can be left to infuse the clothes while they are in the drawers or closets. Put a drop on little cotton ball and place it between the clothes

Clothes Sweeter

- Lemon - 4 drops

- Geranium – 2 drops

- Bois de rose - 3 drops

Mix all essential oils and take a drop on little cotton ball and put it between the clothes.

Moths Repellants

To keep moths away from your clothes use 2-3 drops of one of the following oils. These are particularly useful when coats and woolen are stored away during the summer months.

- Lavender
- Lemon grass
- Rosemary
- Citronella

Essential Oil Blends for Bed Room

Blend 1

- Rose - 10 drops

- Jasmine - 8 drops

- Palmarosa - 7 drops

- Clary sage - 3 drops

Mix all oils into 60 ml of water into the spray bottle. Spray it in the air and on the carpet.

Blend 2

- Palmarosa - 10 drops

- Lime - 8 drops

- Nutmeg - 4 drops

- Ylang ylang - 2 drops

- Cleary sage - 4 drops

Combine the essential oils into the diffuser and turn it on. A diffuser will help you to sleep.

Chapter Nineteen: Recommended for Further Study and Recipe Experimentation

As with anything worth doing, using aromatherapy in a proficient manner takes many years of practicing, researching and experimenting. To help you in expanding your education and experiences, I recommend you visit the following websites:

The American Academy of Neurological and Orthopaedic Surgeons:

http://www.aanos.org/jrl_an_article.htm

Easy Aromatherapy Recipes:

http://www.easy-aromatherapy-recipes.com/

Massage Today:

http://www.massagetoday.com/archives/200 5/02/08.html

National Association of Holistic Aromatherapy:

http://www.naha.org/articles/How%20To%20Use%20Essential%20Oils%20Effectively.htm and http://www.naha.org/explore-aromatherapy/safety/

University of Minnesota:

http://www.takingcharge.csh.umn.edu/explore-healing-practices/aromatherapy/how-do-i-choose-and-use-essential-oils

There are countless websites and books worthy of visiting and reading to mention all of them in this list. Nevertheless, I do highly encourage you to go online and do a more thorough investigation of essential oils. I also highly recommend that you go to a library and check out books on essential oils, botany, Bach flower remedies and aromatherapy. Fortunately, you do not have to know each of the 700+ essential oils thoroughly. You just have to know which essential oils work best for you in each of the areas that essential oils provide benefits. Become familiar with a few oils in each of these therapeutic categories and you will be all set to start mixing your own blends.

Conclusion

Moreover, I greatly encourage you to do more research on olfactory stimuli and their impact. As you should have inferred from all the information imparted in these pages, there is quite a lot more to learn about the human sense of smell and its effects on our daily lives. So go forth and bravely explore where no human has gone before! Go follow your nose and see what adventures it leads you on. Just remember to use a practical approach to aromatherapy and essential oils wherever that venture takes you.